THE

SOUTHERN GARDENER

AND

RECEIPT-BOOK,

CONTAINING

VALUABLE INFORMATION, ORIGINAL AND OTHERWISE,

ON ALL SUBJECTS CONNECTED WITH

DOMESTIC AND RURAL AFFAIRS,

GARDENING, COOKERY, BEVERAGES, DAIRY, MEDICAL,

VETERINARY AND MISCELLANEOUS.

THIRD EDITION,

REVISED AND CORRECTED BY

MRS. MARY L. EDGEWORTH.

PHILADELPHIA:

J. B. LIPPINCOTT & CO.

1860.

THIS VOLUME

Is Affectionately Dedicated

TO

MRS. ELIZABETH THORNTON,

OF

CAMDEN, SOUTH CAROLINA,

AS A

MARK OF ESTEEM FOR HER EXALTED WORTH

IN ALL THE RELATIONS OF LIFE.

M. L. E.

PREFACE

TO THE THIRD EDITION.

THE general favor with which the first two editions of this book were received by the public; the very frequent demands for it since all the copies have been disposed of; together with the numerous solicitations of my friends for its republication, have induced me to undertake a task which, I trust, will prove as valuable to others as it has been agreeable to me.

To the present edition are added many original receipts, as well as some that have been carefully selected; all of which, together with those in the former editions, have been thoroughly tested, and their value well ascertained.

The aim of the author has been to present to the public, in a plain, concise and accessible form, information on all subjects appertaining to domestic and rural affairs, avoiding, as far as possible, technical language. Although the gatherings from a field so extensive must necessarily be numerous, yet the whole has been so systematically classed, and each subject so arranged under its appropriate head, that the desired information may be found without trouble. Those receipts which could not, with propriety, be elsewhere arranged, have been placed under the head of MISCELLANEOUS.

The directions for GARDENING were written expressly for this work by Mr. PHINEAS THORNTON, of Camden, South Carolina, well known as one of the best gardeners of the South. Having been engaged in the business about forty years, his long experience, faithfully recorded, cannot be otherwise than valuable. These directions are not, as the title would indicate, limited in their usefulness to the South only; but, on the contrary, will prove equally applicable to all sections of our country, with some little variation in time, dependent on latitude or climate.

For the MEDICAL department, prescriptions and receipts have been collected from the most reliable sources. My husband (a practising physician) has contributed a number of prescriptions for special diseases, which, from several years' successful use, can be confidently recommended.

In the department of COOKERY, much pains has been taken in proportioning the recipes, so as to adapt them to the tastes, requirements and means of all. Since so much of health, happiness and domestic comfort depends upon the proper preparation of our daily food, it should be the pride and pleasure of every housekeeper to cook well. To assist in acquiring this skill, something new will be found in this book.

MARY L. EDGEWORTH.

FORT VALLEY,
Houston County,
Georgia.

CONTENTS.

For complete Alphabetical Index, see end of the Volume.

THE

SOUTHERN GARDENER

AND

RECEIPT BOOK.

GARDENING.

TO CHOOSE THE BEST SOIL FOR A GARDEN.

PREFER a sandy loam, not less than two feet deep, and good earth, not of a binding nature in summer, nor retentive of rain in winter; but of such a texture, that it can be worked without difficulty at any season of the year. There are few sorts of fruit-trees, or esculent vegetables, which require less depth of earth to grow in than two feet, to bring them to perfection, and if the earth of the kitchen-garden be three or more feet deep, so much the better; for where the plants are in a state of maturity, if the roots, even of peas, spinach, kidney-beans, lettuce, &c., be minutely traced, they will be found to penetrate into the earth, in search of food, to the depth of two feet, provided the soil be of a nature that allows them. If it can be done, a garden should be made on land the bottom of which is not of a springy, wet nature. If this rule can be observed, draining will be unnecessary, for when land is well prepared for the growth of fruit-trees and esculent vegetables, by trenching, manuring, and digging, it is by these means brought into such a porous temperament, that rain passes through without being detained longer than is necessary. When land is of too strong a nature, it should be well mixed with gravel and sand.

TO PREPARE HOT-BEDS, MANURES AND COMPOSTS.

Stable manure is in the most general use for forming hot-beds — which are masses of this manure after it has undergone its violent fermentation. Leaves, especially oak-leaves, when perfectly decayed, form a rich mould, or excellent manure. The object of preparation in these substances, is to get rid of the violent heat produced when the fermentation is going on. It is obvious that *that* preparation must consist in facilitating the process.

For this purpose a certain degree of moisture and air in the fermenting bodies is requisite; and hence the business of the gardener is, to turn them over frequently, and apply water, when the process appears impeded, and exclude rain, when chilled with too much water. Stable manure requires to lie a month or longer in ridges or beds, and to be turned over in that time thrice, before it is fit for cucumber beds of common construction. Tan bark and leaves require a month also.

Fermentation is always more rapid in summer; and if the materials are spread abroad during frost, it is totally impeded. Ashes are often used with manure, and promote the steadiness and duration of their heat.

SOWING SEED.

The usual cause of seed not growing, is owing to their not being well rolled or pressed. When sowing on a large scale, rolling would be more expeditious; but for small sowings, the following may answer as a substitute:—

After the seed is sown, and the ground raked evenly, take a board of the length of the bed; lay it flat on the ground, and walk the whole length of the board. This will press the soil on the seed. Then shift the board till you have thus gone over the whole bed. In dry, warm weather, cover your seed-beds for two or three days with boards laid flat on the soil, or green pine boughs, taking care to remove them at night that the beds may have air and the night dew. By this method the seed will soon vegetate and grow. Late in the spring, or during summer, seed should not be sown or planted, unless there be a good season of rain, or the ground be sufficiently moist. In a dry time the ground might be well watered over night, and sow or plant the following morning. In this case the seed should be previously soaked in soft rain-water from twelve to forty-eight hours, particularly beets, as they are difficult to get up when sown late in the season, on account of their hard shell or covering. Therefore they should have forty-eight hours' soaking, letting them stand in the sun to keep the water warm. Parsnips or carrots might be soaked the same length of time.

GERMINATION OF GARDEN SEED.

M. Humboldt has made several experiments on the subject of the germination of seed in the oxymuriatic acid, or oxalic acid diluted with water, and has found that this acid has a remarkable effect in accelerating the progress of vegetation. Cress seed, when thrown into this fluid at the temperature of 88°, showed germs in three hours, while none were seen in water in twenty-six hours. Professor Pohl, at Dresden, produced in this manner vegetation from dried seed one hundred years old; and Messrs. Jacquere and Vanden Schott, at Vienna, have caused the growth of old seed in the botanical garden, which have resisted every other method.

VEGETATION OF GARDEN SEED.

The number of years during which different Garden Seed will retain the vegetative principle.

	YEARS.		YEARS.		YEARS.
Artichoke	3	Endive	4	Potato	3
Asparagus	4	Fennel	5	Pumpkin	10
Balm	2	Garlic	3	Purslain	2
Basil	2	Gourd	10	Radish	2
Bean	1	Hop	2	Rampion	2
Beet	10	Horseradish	4	Rape	4
Borage	4	Hyssop	6	Rhubarb	1
Broccoli	4	Jerusalem Artichoke	3	Rosemary	3
Burnet	6	Lavender	2	Rue	3
Cabbage	4	Leek	2	Ruta Baga	4
Camomile	2	Lettuce	3	Salsify	2
Caraway	4	Marigold	2	Samphire	3
Carrot	1	Melon	10	Summer Savory	2
Cauliflower	4	Mint	4	Scorzenera	2
Celery	10	Mustard	4	Shalot	4
Chervil	6	Mangel Wurzel	10	Sherret	4
Cives	3	Marjoram	4	Sorrel	7
Corn	3	Nasturtion	2	Spinach	4
Corn Salad	2	Onion	2	Squash	10
Coriander	3	Parsley	6	Tansy	3
Cress	2	Pea	1	Thyme	2
Cucumber	10	Parsnip	1	Tomato	2
Dandelion	10	Pennyroyal	2	Turnip	6
Dock	1			Wormwood	2

TO SAVE SEEDS.

All seeds save better in their seed-vessels, but this can rarely be done, on account of the great space occupied. As soon therefore as the pods of cabbages, turnips, radishes, &c., turn brown and a part become dry, the stems should be cut and laid on a cloth or floor to dry, afterwards threshed out and hung up in bags in a dry room.

ASPARAGUS

May be sown any time during the month of March, in a small bed of light, rich soil, drilled in rows nine inches apart, which would be preferable to broad-cast, on account of hoeing and keeping them clear of weeds, covering them one inch deep; should the weather prove dry, water them occasionally. In twelve months (or say in the month of February, after the plants are up), they may be set out in beds six feet wide, by twenty-five or thirty feet in length, with walks two-and-a-half feet wide between each bed, sufficient to admit a wheelbarrow. The beds are previously prepared by spading to the depth of twelve or fifteen inches. After the bed is leveled and raked fine, proceed to lay it off in trenches, across the bed, two feet apart from each other, each trench to be dug fifteen inches wide and two-and-a-half feet deep, laying up the soil in ridges between each trench. Should the natural soil not be good to that depth, the inferior at the bottom may be removed and carried off: after this is done, throw in eighteen inches of well-rotted stable manure; after leveling the same, add two inches of soil on the manure, taken from the sides which were thrown out of the ridges; level this also and rake it finely, and all is ready for planting.

Then be careful in selecting such plants only as have good fiber, and a fine bold crown; in setting out, place them eighteen inches apart, and lay out the fiber in regular order, and not tumble them together, as is too often done, to the great injury of the plants. When this is done, cover them with two inches more of the soil from the sides of the ridges, as before, and the work is done. Plants eighteen months or two years old would be preferable, as they would be more vigorous. The plants throughout the summer must be kept clear of weeds, and occasionally hoed, and the loose dirt gradually thrown in from the sides of the ridges. By these operations, and the summer rains, the trenches will by October be filled up as level as the bed was before setting out the roots. Upon the approach of cold weather, and after the tops have been killed by frost, they should be cut down even with the ground and carried off; the bed should then be covered with two or three inches of coarse stable manure, partly rotten, which should remain on the bed until spring, when it must be forked, or hoed carefully into the surface of the bed so as not to injure the crowns of the roots. Just before the shoots make their appearance in the spring, the beds should be carefully raked free from weeds.

No kind of vegetable seed should be sown in the beds between the plants, as it exhausts the goodness of the soil. The first year after planting the bed, a few of the strongest shoots may be cut, but it should be sparingly, as the roots will be all the better afterward. Continue to pursue the same system of culture every year, and the roots will rapidly increase in vigor. Beds prepared in this manner, and yearly attended to, will last many years, and the produce will be of a superior quality. Asparagus thrives in a light, rich soil, neither too wet nor too dry. There are two or three varieties of this plant, but the giant asparagus is the largest and most productive. By analysis it is ascertained that the elements of asparagus are mainly supplied by bone manure and superphosphate of lime.

ARTICHOKE.

This is a perennial plant, a fine vegetable for table use, and highly esteemed by many. There are two or three varieties. The largest globe has a dusky, purplish head; the dwarfish globe is a prolific variety, and valuable as occupying less room with its head. They are propagated by suckers, or by seed. The seed may be sown any time during the month of March, in small beds of tolerably light, good soil, drilled in rows twelve inches apart. In order to procure good thrifty plants, the seed should be dropped singly nine or ten inches apart, and covered two inches deep; work them occasionally, keeping the ground loose and light, and free from weeds. About the last of August, or early in September, the plants may be set out in large beds of a deep, rich, light soil, moist but not wet, giving the plants three feet space each way, being careful that the hearts do not get covered with the earth. It would be well to have the beds situated so as to have a gentle slope, sufficient to carry off any superfluous moisture or water that might accumulate during the winter or spring. If the slope of the beds were to face the south, it might hasten the vegetation of the plants so as to produce heads for use the following summer. Late in the fall, or about the last of November, when vegetation has ceased, the dead leaves may be removed from the plants, and the beds covered with a good coat of manure from the stable, partly rotten, with fine straw, or other coarse litter, to the depth of two or three inches, observing that the plants be lightly covered. Bone dust and wood ashes also improve the soil. In the spring, before the plants begin to vegetate, the beds may be lightly spaded, or hoed, so as not to injure the plants, and raked finely afterward, in order to destroy all superfluous weeds. The ground should be worked occasionally during the spring and summer, so as to be kept light and loose, and free from weeds. By the above mode and treatment, the plants will bear and do well for six or seven years. After the plants have been bearing two years, the stocks may be examined in the spring (say the last of February), and two or three of the strongest or best shoots being selected for growing, the rest are removed with a knife or chisel. These shoots or suckers may be transplanted into new beds, as before described. When all the heads from a stem are taken, cut off the stem close to the ground, to give the plant more strength for new shoots.

The plant called Jerusalem artichoke is not properly an artichoke, and would not be ranked as a vegetable for the table. Its root, which is similar to a potato, contains but very little nutriment, therefore is but of little value. The growth of the plant or stalk resembles the sunflower, and is of the easiest possible cultivation; will grow in almost any soil, and when it has once got possession of the ground it is very difficult to eradicate: as hogs will eat them, they are sometimes cultivated for that purpose. For a crop, they may be planted after the ground is well ploughed, any time in March, in drills two and a half or three feet apart, and may be planted and worked as corn crops, hilling them a little when worked with a hoe. They may be cut in two or three pieces like potatoes, and dropped in the drills twelve inches apart, and covered two or three inches deep. They will produce more abundantly in a strong, light clay soil. As the root is firm and hard, they are sometimes made use of for pickles.

BEETS

May be sown the last of February, or early in March, and in order for a succession of crops, they may be sown till the last of April, in beds prepared of a light, strong, rich soil, and spaded to the depth of twelve or fifteen inches, and made four or five feet wide. After the beds are leveled and raked finely, they may be drilled in rows, twenty inches apart. The seed may be dropped singly five or six inches apart, and covered two inches deep. As the plants will admit, thin out to stand singly twelve or fifteen inches apart. In order to have large thrifty plants, the ground should be frequently worked, and made very light and loose, and kept free from weeds. Should the fall season prove favorable by not being dry, they might be sown from the first to the tenth of August, and come to perfection before the winter sets in; but the early sowing is most favorable to this climate. Beets sown in a light, dry soil, after the month of March, should be soaked thirty-six hours, and kept in the sun in the course of the day, to keep the water warm; after the seed is sown and raked in, the ground should be well pressed. When the beets have their full growth, which may be noted by their tops being decayed or dead, they may be dug up, and preserved by being packed away in light, dry sand, either in boxes or barrels. It would be well to spread them on the ground for a day or two, in the shade, to give them air to evaporate the surplus moisture. Prepare the soil the autumn before planting with common salt and unleached ashes.

BEANS.

Bush beans of all descriptions, if the spring be favorable, may be planted the first of April, and in order for a succession of crops, they should be planted once in two or three weeks till the last of May, in a light, rich soil, in trenches from two to two-and-a-half feet apart, covered two inches; and when the plants will admit, hoe and thin them out to stand four or five inches apart. Bush beans, for a full crop, may be planted from the fifteenth of July to the twentieth of August. Pole beans, of all descriptions, may be planted from the fifth of April to the last of May, in drills from three to five feet apart, according to the height they run; and as the plants will admit, thin them out to stand from nine to twelve inches apart. Two beans or vines may be admitted to run to one pole. Sometimes they are planted in hills from three to four feet apart each way, and three or four beans may be planted in a hill, but only two thrifty vines left to run to one pole. Those kinds which do not run so much, may be planted with corn when about six inches in height, and if the soil be light and strong, will do well; but when this method is adopted, the corn should be planted in drills or trenches from four to five feet apart, and the corn thinned out, leaving a space of two feet between each stalk. Then plant two or three to each stalk, leaving only two or three thrifty plants to run. Lima beans might be planted with advantage in a single row, along a border on each side of a walk, and poles might be bent over in the form of an arch for them to run on. By this means they might be easily gathered when grown. They are one of the best kind of shell beans for table use, and require a good, strong, light soil. They will bear till frost, and will stand the dry weather much better than any other kind, and are, therefore, the most profitable crop. They may be gathered in the fall, after they become dry, and laid away for winter use. By soaking them in soft water over-night, previous to cooking them, they will boil very sweet and tender, and are very fine for soup. As they are more tender than other varieties, they should not be planted sooner than the tenth or fifteenth of April. Windsor beans are one of those varieties that are very hardy, and will stand the winter frost For early spring use, they may be planted from the first to the middle of October, in a strong, rich soil, in trenches from two and a half to three feet apart, and covered three inches deep; and when the plants will admit, they may be thinned out so as to stand from six to eight inches apart, and for a succession of crops they might be planted again the last of February and early in March. Wood-ashes and bone-dust, or superphosphate of lime, are suitable fertilizers.

BORECOLE

Is a species of cabbage, and one of those hardy plants, the leaves of which may be cut without injury to its growth, and will produce a new crop in the course of a month or six weeks. They may be sown in small beds, made light and loose, about the last of February, or any time during the month of March, in drills nine inches apart, and covered one inch deep. In order to have good, thrifty plants, and of a regular size, thin them out a little soon after they are up, and in a few days more thin them ont again, so as to give the plants three or four inches space; and when the plants will admit, they may be set out in beds or squares previously dug, and made light and loose, at the distance of two-and-a-half feet apart each way. It should be observed that the land must be well manured, and in a high state of tillage, for the cultivation of this plant, which, if kept constantly hoed, will grow very luxuriantly, and in the hottest weather be infinitely more brittle in the leaves than any other kind cultivated in gardens, which is a certain indication of its being a healthy plant. It is worthy of the attention of the farmer or grazier on occount of the rapidity of its growth and the property of withstanding the effect of severe frost, while it affords an excellent vegetable for the table, and may be used with advantage for feeding cows and sheep. There are several species of this plant, but the green curled borecole is the hardiest and best.

BROCCOLI.

A species of cabbage cultivated for the use of the table. There are several kinds of this plant, but the purple Cape Broccoli is said to be the best. It may be sown about the latter end of February or early in March, in any tolerable soil, in drills eight or nine inches apart, and covered one inch deep; and when plants have germinated eight leaves, they should be transplanted into nursery beds, in rows twelve inches apart, and the plants five or six inches from each other. By this means the plants would have a more regular, stout growth. Should the weather prove dry, they might be frequently watered, which should be done at night, observing to stir the ground loose around the plants the following morning; and in order to make them flourish and grow, they should be kept in a good state of tillage, and free from weeds during the whole growth. About the first of May they may be set out in large beds of a light, strong soil, and well sheltered, or where the shade would strike them early in the day, giving them a few hours of the early morning sun: give the plants two feet space from each other. As our summers frequently prove too hot and dry for the early sowing and planting of this vegetable to mature and come to perfection, they might be sown about the middle of July, on shady beds or borders, and watered occasionally should the weather prove dry, observing when the plants are well up to thin them out six or eight inches apart, to give them a good regular growth; and about the middle of August they might be set out in beds, as above described. They would then be apt to flower and head well before the hard weather set in. Should the winter prove mild, they would continue to head and put out during the winter season. Broccoli requires the same manures as cabbage.

CAULIFLOWER.

The early cauliflower may be sown from the tenth to the last of February, in any tolerable soil, in drills six inches apart, and covered one inch deep: and when they produce three leaves they may be put into nursery beds, as the broccoli, and about the last of April set out or transplanted, where they may remain, giving them a good, light soil. The late cauliflower may be sown about the last of April, and set out in nursery beds as above; and about the last of June, may be set out where they are to remain, giving them a space of two feet each way. Those that are headed must have the heads shaded by breaking the large leaves over them.

CARROTS.

For summer use, may be sown from the middle of February to the last of March, in beds prepared four feet wide, of a light, rich soil, drilled in rows twelve inches apart, and covered one inch deep. As soon as the plants are well up, they may be thinned out, to stand one or two inches apart, and as they advance a little in size, thin them out to stand three or four inches from each other. By this mode, and frequently stirring the ground finely, the roots will be of a regular and good size. For winter and spring use, carrots may be sown from the first to the last of August, and treated as above.

Carrots should not be sown late in the spring, and early in the fall, unless there be a good season of rain, observing to roll or press the ground after the seeds are raked in. The salt and lime mixture, composted with leaf-mould, a little plaster of Paris, bone-dust, and wood-ashes, are the special manures.

EARLY CABBAGE

May be sown the last of January, or early in February, in warm beds of any tolerably light soil, either in broad-cast, or in drills nine inches apart, which would be preferàble, on account of hoeing and keeping them free from weeds: cover them one inch deep, and when the plants are well up, they may be thinned out to stand two or three inches apart. By this means they will be more thrifty, and regular in size. When the plants will admit, they may be set out in beds of rich mould, previously made loose and light, each plant two feet apart.

Late cabbage may be sown the last of May, or any time in June, and remain in the beds till August before transplanting, and may be set out in the same manner as the early ones.

Green glazed cabbage may be sown any time in February or March, and treated as the others, only giving them a little more space when transplanted. Early cabbage, sown from the twentieth of September, to the first of October, on a warm border, would produce heads two or three weeks earlier, should the winter prove favorable, and not too severe.

RAISING CABBAGE FROM CUTTINGS.

A neighbor of ours tells us, that he, accidentally, raised some fine cabbage from cuttings last year. Some pieces of old stumps happened to be buried in the spring, at the proper depth. They soon sent up shoots (one each) at an early day, and formed excellent heads. There was no tendency to seed, any more than from plants obtained in the usual way.

To try the experiment of getting early cabbage in this way, cut the stump into small pieces, with one bud on each; plant and cultivate them as you would plants from the seed.

TO KILL LICE ON CABBAGE.

Last year I had one quarter of an acre of cabbage that were nearly covered with the cabbage-louse. I took off the outside leaves, and burned them. Having a few gallons of very strong tobacco liquor (left after sheep-shearing,) which I diluted by adding soap-suds from the wash, I sprinkled the plants very thoroughly from a watering-pot. I believe it killed every louse, for I did not discover one afterwards.

TO DESTROY WORMS ON CABBAGE.

Tobacco-leaves strewn upon and among cabbage are said to be effectual in preventing the ravages of cabbage-worms.

SOLID CELERY

May be sown in March, on a small bed of light rich soil, in drills six or nine inches apart, and covered lightly. When the plants are up to the height of an inch or two, they may be thinned out to stand three or four inches apart, so as to give them a regular, good growth. Should the weather prove dry, the plants may be occasionally watered at night, observing to stir the ground between the plants the following morning. When the plants are from six to nine inches in height, and have acquired a stocky growth, they may be set out in a very rich, moist soil, previously prepared, in trenches three feet apart and a spade deep: lay the earth on each side of the trenches, and dig the bottom, leaving them level: place the plants along the trenches upright six inches apart, and water them, should the weather prove dry afterwards; they might be shaded in the day for two or three days till they have taken root. In three or four weeks draw the earth to each side of the plants, breaking it fine: do this in dry weather, and be careful not to bury the hearts: repeat the earthing once in ten or twelve days till the plants are fit for use. In order for a succession of crops they may be sown in April and May, and treated as above. Seeds sown later than April should be sown in a moist, shady situation, and the ground well pressed. As they are sometimes difficult to get up when sown late, it might be well to water the beds for three or four evenings, should the weather prove dry, and cover them in the day with green pine boughs. Salt and ashes would be a good manure.

CURLED CRESS, OR PEPPERGRASS,

May be sown the last of March, or early in April, in beds of a tolerably good soil, in drills six inches apart, and covered lightly; and in order for a succession of crops it may be sown once in two or three weeks, till the last of May.

Garden cress may be sown as above, only give it nine inches space between the drills, and as soon as well up thin them out so that the plants may stand single two or three inches apart.

CUCUMBERS,

For early use, may be planted about the first of April, in a good, warm, light soil: should the nights prove cool about the time they should come up, or after, the hills may be covered with straw at night, and removed in the day, when the sun is up, so as to warm the hills. For a succession of crops, the long green may be planted for pickling the last of May, and early in June, in a moist soil, so it be light and good; the early sort in hills four feet apart each way; and the long green, or late sort, in hills six feet apart each way, leaving only one thrifty plant in a hill to grow. Put no fresh manure in the hills, as it is too powerful, and will cause them to wilt and die. If the soil be light and poor, make up hills about two feet square, by throwing out the soil to the depth of fifteen or eighteen inches; then fill up the hole with good rich mould, well pulverized: a little of the top soil first taken off might be mixed with the mould near the top, observing to leave the hill only a little above the level of the ground. In order that they may be kept in a flourishing state, and bear till late, the ground must be kept loose and free from weeds, and no cucumber suffered to remain on the vine till full grown, except such as are wanted for seed. Should the weather prove very dry, they might be occasionally watered at night, by filling a small trench — made before the vines commence running — with water, that it may run to the roots. This is preferable to sprinkling water on the tops of the hills, or plants, as the vines are very tender. The seeds should not be planted till the ground is warm; they will then come up quick, and grow without any obstruction; otherwise, if they come up, and get stunted by the cold, they do not flourish well afterwards. For a fall crop for pickling, they might be planted the last of July, and early in August. To save cucumbers from the streaked bug, plant an onion in each hill.

When cucumbers are planted later than the month of April, it would be well to spread a coat of fine straw on the ground between the hills, to the depth of three or four inches, immediately after a rain.

By this method they would not suffer by the drought; and if the season prove wet, the vines will not be so liable to rot.

NOVEL METHOD OF RAISING CUCUMBERS.

After all that the doctors have said against cucumbers, they are still a welcome dish upon most tables, and, when eaten in moderation, are probably healthful. That they are not so when eaten immoderately, is, we have no doubt, also true. Cucumbers are most sought after early in the season, and we will now proceed to tell how we managed last year to have them in perfection long before they were plentiful in market.

Having cleared the soil to the depth of twelve or fifteen inches from a space four feet in diameter, we placed an old nail-keg in the centre, and filled up around with fresh manure, and covered it over with six or eight inches of earth, forming a mound of a foot or more in height, and six feet in diameter, with the open-ended keg in the centre, into which in very dry weather we could pour water, which would escape into the manure through the openings, and prevent the perishing of the vines. The seeds were planted in the mound (not in the keg, for that was empty) in March or in April, and the heat of the fermenting manure forced them vigorously. We had heavy frost afterward, and the surface of the earth was completely frozen; but it was only necessary to lay a board over the plants, and the warmth below was amply sufficient to protect them. The only object in using the keg was to prevent the water from running off and forming gutters down the sides of the mound. The plan worked well, and as it may be advantageous to others also, we publish it for the general benefit. A frame for the vines to run upon is advantageous.

EGG PLANT

May be sown on a warm border about the first of April, in drills nine inches apart, and covered one inch deep; and where the plants will admit, they may be set out in beds of a light, rich soil, giving them two feet space each way between the plants; hoe, and keep them free from weeds, and as they advance in size draw a little earth around the stems. There are two varieties of this plant, the white and the purple: the latter is preferable for table use; the white is more for ornament, as the growth is not so large. The plants may be set out eighteen inches apart. They make a handsome ornament for the flower-pot.

GHERKINS

May be planted from the middle of April to the last of May, in any tolerable soil, so that it is light and warm, in hills six or eight feet apart, leaving but one thrifty plant in a hill to grow. If they be kept free from weeds, and the summer is moderately dry, they will bear abundantly till frost. They are very fine for pickles.

GOURDS

May be planted from the first to the last of April, in a good, light, rich soil, in hills six or eight feet apart. And the mammoth gourd may be planted from the middle of March to the last of April, in hills from eight to ten feet apart.

KAIL,

For early spring greens, may be sown about the last of January, in small beds of a light, rich soil, in drills twelve inches apart, and covered one inch deep. As soon as the plants are well up, thin them out to stand two or three inches apart: afterward they may be thinned out for use as they advance in size: those that remain for seed should have fifteen or eighteen inches space.

LETTUCE,

For early use, may be sown the last of January on warm borders of a light, rich soil, prepared well and raked fine, in drills nine inches apart, and covered lightly; and in order that the plants may be fine, and of a regular size, thin them out as soon as they are well up, to stand three or four inches apart; stir the ground frequently, and keep them free from weeds. As soon as the plants will admit, set them out in beds, or round the borders, fifteen inches apart; if the ground be very rich and light, they will head well. In order for a succession they may be sown once in three or four weeks till the last of April. Wood-ashes, common salt and animal manure will improve the soil.

LAVENDER, SAGE, BALM, TANSY, THYME, RUE, ROSEMARY OR OTHER HERBS,

May be sown by the last of March, or early in April, in small beds made light and fine, and drilled in rows nine inches apart, and covered one inch deep. When the plants will admit, they may be thinned out, to stand four or five inches apart: in the following winter, say in January or February, they may be set out in small beds, each plant from eighteen inches to two feet apart, according to the size they grow.

MUSTARD,

For winter use, may be sown from the middle of September to the middle of October, on warm borders of a tolerably rich, light soil, and covered lightly in drills fifteen inches apart; for spring use, it may be sown again from the middle to the last of February, in beds spaded and well prepared, in drills eighteen inches apart. In order that the plants may flourish and grow quick, thin them out as soon as they are well up, to stand two or three inches apart. Afterwards they may be thinned out as wanted for use. Those that are to remain for seed should be thinned out to stand twelve or fifteen inches apart.

NASTURTIONS

May be sown the last of March, or early in April, in a very light, rich soil, in drills four feet apart; drop the seeds three or four inches apart, and cover them two inches deep: when the plants will admit, thin them out, to stand nine inches apart. The plants should be supported from the ground by bushy sticks. Should the spring be dry, they should be occasionally watered in the evening, observing to stir the ground around the roots loosely the following morning. In a warm climate they would flourish best planted on a shady border, where the shade would strike them early in the day. The leaves, as well as the fruit, are sometimes used for pickles. As it is very ornamental, they might be planted in boxes, with a light, rich soil, one seed in a box, and watered every evening till they come up, and placed on a shelf on the shady side of the house. They should be watered every evening, if the weather be dry, and the ground loosened around the plant the following morning. By this method the plants will grow very luxuriantly.

OKRA

May be planted any time in the month of April, in a large bed of light, rich soil, drilled in rows four feet apart, and covered one inch deep. When the plants will admit, thin them out, to stand one-and-a-half or two feet apart, according to the strength of the ground. If the okra be planted in drills, six feet apart, cucumbers might be planted in hills between the rows, and do very well.

MODE OF RAISING ONIONS IN THE TOWN OF WETHERSFIELD, CONNECTICUT.

The town of Wethersfield has long been famous for the large quantities of onions which are annually raised, and exported to the West Indies and the southern States. It has been superstitiously supposed that there is something in the soil of Wethersfield peculiarly adapted to the culture of onions; and this whim has, no doubt, discouraged many from attempting the cultivation of this valuable root in other sections of the country equally favorable to its growth. It is true the soil of Wethersfield is a rich, sandy loam, well adapted to horticultural purposes; but the success of its inhabitants in the cultivation of onions, is attributable in a much greater degree to a particular virtue in the fingers of its females, than any peculiar properties of its soil.

The business of raising onions in Wethersfield is reduced to a perfect system. The following is the method of cultivation: Early in the spring, the land is manured by ploughing in fine manure from the stable or barn-yard, in the proportion of about ten loads to the acre. That of neat cattle is preferred, as that of horses is considered of too heating a nature. Ashes, bone-dust and the salt and lime mixture are also good fertilizers. After the manure is ploughed in, the land is well harrowed and laid out in beds five feet wide.

The beds are laid out by turning a furrow toward them each way. This raises the bed above the aisles, and gives an opportunity for the water to run off, should there be occasion for it. They are then raked with an iron tooth or common hay-rake, and the aisles suffered to remain as left by the plough. Thus prepared, the beds are ready to receive the seed.

As early as the season will admit, the seed is sown in the following manner: a rake with teeth a foot apart is drawn crosswise to the beds, for the purpose of making drills for the reception of the seeds. The seed is then sown in the drills with the thumb and fingers, and covered with the hand. From ten to twelve pounds of seed are put upon an acre. After the plants come up they are kept free from weeds, which generally requires four weedings; a hoe of suitable width to pass between the rows is used in weeding, which saves much labor. When ripe, they are pulled, and the tops cut off with a knife. A sufficient length of top is left to tie them to the straw in roping, or in bunches of three and a half pounds, as required by a law of the State. An ordinary crop is from six thousand to eight thousand ropes to the acre. The quantity annually raised in the town is estimated from one million to two millions and a half of ropes, which are sold at an average price of two dollars a hundred, amounting to from twenty to thirty thousand dollars.

Most of the labor of raising onions in Wethersfield is performed by females. The cultivation of an acre requires from fifty to sixty days' labor of a female, whose rate of wages, including board, is about forty-two cents a day. Though many of the young ladies of Wethersfield spend a portion of their time in their onion gardens, yet in personal beauty, education, and politeness, they are not excelled by most females of far less industrious habits.

LEEKS

May be sown early in September on a warm border open to the south, in drills nine inches apart, and covered lightly. About the middle of February following, the plants may be drawn up and set out in beds of four or five feet wide, previously prepared by spading in rich manure well rotted and pulverized, and the beds may be laid off in trenches of four or five inches deep, and fifteen inches apart. Make holes with a dibble three inches deep at the bottom of the trench, and six inches apart, to receive the roots. A portion of the straggling roots and tops may be cropped or cut off; when the plants are set, close the dirt lightly around the roots, leave the trench open, and draw up the earth to the plants as they grow till the trenches are made level. By this method the roots will be fine and well blanched.

PARSNIPS

May be sown about the last of February, or any time during the month of March, in beds prepared four feet wide, of a very rich, light earth, dug at least a full spade deep, and drilled in rows eighteen inches apart, and covered one inch deep. When the plants will admit, they may be thinned out to stand twelve or fifteen inches apart. Cabbage-seed may be drilled between each row, and do well, as the cabbages would be remvoed before they would prove an injury to the parsnips. Peppergrass might also be sown in drills between the parsnips, and would prove no injury, as it is made use off as salads, or rather used with lettuce, and would be removed before the parsnips got to be of any size.

As parsnips, carrots, and beets, are difficult seed to get up when sown late, they should not be sown after the month of March, without a good season of rain, soaking the parsnips and carrots from twenty-four to thirty-six hours, and the beets forty-eight hours before planting, either in warm water or letting it stand in the sun, which will answer the purpose, observing to press the ground well after the seed is sown and raked in; and if the soil is light and dry, it would be well, after the seed is raked in, to cover the bed a few days with plank or green pine bushes, observing to remore them at night to give the beds air, and to have the advantage of the night dews. By this method they will not fail to come up, if the seed is good. Potash and phosphoric acid are the elements most likely to be wanting in the soil. Apply wood-ashes and bone-dust.

PARSLEY

May be sown early in February, but would do best sown in September, in small beds of a good, light soil, in drills six inches apart, and covered one inch deep.

As soon as the plants will admit, thin them out to stand three or four inches apart. As parsley-seed seldom vegetates under five or six weeks, it would be best to give it rather a shady border; and if sown after February, it would be advisable to soak the seed twelve hours in water, mixed with sulphur, observing to press the ground well after the seed is raked in; and should the weather prove dry afterwards, occasionally water the bed. By this method it would soon vegetate and come up.

PEPPERS

May be sown from the tenth to the last of April, in small beds of a light, rich soil, thinly, in drills fifteen to eighteen inches apart, and covered one inch deep. As soon as the plants will admit, thin them out to stand twelve inches apart. Those plants that are drawn out may be transplanted into large beds, of a strong, rich soil, giving them eighteen inches space each way.

ENGLISH PEAS,

For an early spring crop, may be planted any time in December in a light, rich soil, drilled in rows four feet apart, and those that grow very tall require five feet space, covering them two inches deep. As the winter often proves too severe, they might do full as well, or better, planted the last of January, or early in February; and in order for a succession of crops, they may be planted once in three or four weeks after, till the middle of April. They have been proved to do full as well, or better, planted in ridges around the edges or borders of beds, which makes a great saving of ground, and renders the gathering much easier. It is a good plan to plant two rows together, about nine inches apart, so that by setting bushes between them both rows may be held up. The ground should be frequently stirred and made fine around the roots, and kept free from weeds; and, as they advance in height, draw a little earth to the stems. Peas that do not require sticks may be planted in drills two-and-a-half feet apart, or on the edges or borders of beds, as the other kind. Ashes and bone, or superphosphate of lime, are good manures.

RADISHES.

This root being liable to be eaten by worms, the following method is recommended for raising them. Take equal quantities of buckwheat-bran and fresh horse-manure, and mix them well and plentifully, and spread a thick coat on the bed intended for sowing, and spade it in, so that it may get thoroughly mixed. Suddenly after this a great fermentation will be produced, and a number of toadstools (a kind of mushroom) will start up in forty-eight hours. Dig the ground over again, and sow the seeds in drills early in February, and when well up, they may be thinned out, regularly, to stand three or four inches apart, and keep the ground loose and free from weeds. By this method they will grow with great rapidity, and be free from insects. Buckwheat-bran is an excellent manure of itself; also ashes and superphosphate of lime. A second crop of radishes might be raised on the same bed after the first is done, by spading up the ground, and sowing and managing as at first.

RHUBARB, OR PIE PLANT.

This may be propagated either by seed or cuttings: the seeds may be sown on a warm bed early in March, in drills eighteen inches apart, and dropped thinly; and when well up and in a growing state, they may be thinned out, in order to give the plants a good, regular growth, to stand six inches apart. The soil should be kept light and loose around the plants, and free from weeds during the summer: and in the month of September following, the plants may be removed to a stationary bed, previously prepared, of a deep rich mold, well spaded in, the ground inclined to be moist, but not wet. The plants may be set out two-and-a-half feet each way; and, before the cold weather sets in, there may be a coat of half-rotted manure spread over the beds, which will benefit and strengthen the roots. The after management of rhubarb requires good culture, and keeping clean; and every fall the beds should have a good coat of well-rotted manure spread over. As young plants produce the most tender stalks or canes, new beds should be made once in three years, which might be done by dividing the old roots and crowns in such a manner that each set has one or more eyes, and planting in September, as above stated. Rhubarb is remarkable for the quantity of phosphates and soda it extracts from the earth. Crude soda or bone-dust may also be added as a fertilizer.

SALSIFY OR VEGETABLE OYSTER,

Is a white root, resembling a parsnip, and may be sown in small beds, and cultivated in the same manner.

SHALLOTS

May be planted by the middle or the last of February, in drills about fifteen inches apart, laid open three or four inches deep, and in each drill put a sprinkling of salt evenly, and upon that a of dry soot, about half an inch thick; then plant the roots upon it, about six inches apart, and cover up the drill evenly, with the earth firmly round the roots; keep them free from weeds during their growth, and work the ground evenly, without drawing up the earth round the roots. By this method they will produce fine large bulbs.

SPINACH,

For winter use, may be sown the last of September, and again in October; and in order to have a succession of crops for spring use, it may be sown again in February and early in March, in a light strong soil, drilled in rows fifteen inches apart, and covered one inch deep. As soon as the plants are well up, thin them out to stand three or four inches apart; afterward they may be thinned out for use as they advance in size. If any are left to remain for seed, they should have about fifteen inches space.

NEW ZEALAND SPINACH,

A new valuable sort, which may be planted from the twentieth of February to the last of March, in beds prepared, four feet wide, of a good, light, rich mold, in drills twenty inches apart, the seeds dropped singly six inches apart in the drill, and covered nearly two inches deep; and if they should all come up, the plants may be thinned out, to stand eighteen inches apart, and those plants that are taken up will do very well, transplanted in beds as above, giving them the same space. If the ground is well stirred, and the plants kept free from weeds while young, it will spread and be very luxuriant. As it stands the dry hot .her better than almost any other plant, it bears well till frost; as the leaves are plucked off for use, they will put out again.

SUMMER SAVORY

May be sown the last of March, or any time during the month of April, in small beds of almost any tolerable soil, drilled in rows nine inches apart, and covered lightly. Keep the ground loose, and free from weeds, during the growth of the plant.

SPRING TURNIP

May be sown the middle of February for early use, and again till the last of March for a succession, in any tolerably good, light soil, drilled in rows fifteen or eighteen inches apart, and covered one inch deep. As soon as the plants are well up, so as to be able to get hold of them with the fingers, thin them out to stand singly one or two inches apart; and as they advance in size, so as to crowd and touch each other, thin them out again so as to give them three or four inches space: afterwards they may be thinned out for use, giving them a little more space as they advance in size: keep the ground loose and light round the roots, and free from weeds. By this method the turnips will be always well rooted, and the tops very fine. Many persons have said, they never succeed in raising spring turnips, and for that reason have given up the cultivation of them. There are two very good reasons why these people are unsuccessful in their cultivation: one is, that they do not thin them out so as to allow sufficient space; and the next reason is, that they do not sufficiently work the ground, so as to get rid of the weeds. The author of this work has cultivated spring turnips for upwards of thirty years past, and has never failed one spring, when sown early, in having very fine large roots. The common late, flat turnip may be sown from the first of August to the tenth of September, either in broadcast, or drilled in rows as the spring turnip, which would be preferable, in order to work or keep them free from weeds. They should have about eighteen or twenty inches space between the rows, or more, if the ground be strong. The large Norfolk field turnip should have two feet space between the rows, or more, if the ground be strong. New ground, enclosed a year before planting (where cows have used,) is said to be preferable for fall turnips. Previous to sowing, plough it two ways, and run a harrow over it to level and break the ground loose. Hanover turnips may be sown from the twentieth of July to the middle of August: but the early sowing, the last of July or the first of August, will be best, if there should be a good season of rain, as the roots will then have time to get their growth before the winter sets in. They require a strong light soil, either spaded or well ploughed; they may be sown in drills twenty inches or two feet apart, and covered one inch deep. As soon as the plants will admit, thin them, to stand fifteen inches apart; those that are drawn out may be transplanted and do very well.

REMEDY FOR DESTROYING THE TURNIP-FLY.

A remedy for destroying the turnip-fly is to get a quantity of lime from the kilns, in lumps or shells, which, put into a shed, or under cover, and slack it with tobacco water; when it is slacked into a powder, sow it carefully upon the young plants. If any farmer will try this simple remedy, his turnip crop may be saved from the destruction of the fly. Immediately after rain, or while the dew is on the turnip, is the best time for sowing the lime, when it adheres to the leaves of the young plants.

RUTA-BAGA,—QUALITY OF LAND, MANNER OF SOWING, CULTIVATION, &c.

A late fall turnip, has a smooth leaf like a cabbage, and is known in the State of New York by the name of the yellow Russian turnip. There are other varieties similar, which have a leaf of a yellowish green, while the leaf of the ruta-baga is of a bluish green, like the green of peas when nearly full-grown, or like the green of a young and thrifty early York cabbage. The outside of the bulb of the ruta-baga is of a greenish hue, mixed toward the top with a color bordering on a red; and the inside of the bulb, if the sort be true and genuine, is of a deep yellow.

The time of sowing in the State of New York is from the twenty-fifth of June to the tenth of July; but as our seasons here are much longer, and the latter part of the summer generally hot and dry, it would be advisable not to sow sooner than the twentieth of July, and not later than the middle of August.

As a fine, rich garden mold, of a great depth, and having a porous stratum under it, is best for everything that vegetates, except plants that live best in water, so it is best for the ruta-baga. But Cobbett, on the culture of this root, says: "There is no soil in which it may not be cultivated with great facility, except a pure sand, or very stiff clay." A few days previously to sowing, the ground must be plowed into ridges, having two furrows on each side of the ridge, so that every ridge consists of four furrows, or turnings of the plow, making the tops of the ridges nearly, or quite, three feet from each other. As the plowing should be deep, it will of course have a deep gutter between every two ridges. If the ground be not strong, rotten stubble manure may be placed under the middle of each ridge, beneath where the seed is sown. The ground being prepared, lay open a trench in each ridge or row, and sow the seed very thinly, so that they may not touch each other, and cover them one inch deep, observing to press the ground well that the seed may vegetate quickly before the earth gets too dry. This is always a good thing to be done even with any kind of seed that is sown lightly, especially in dry weather and under a hot sun. Seed are very small things. When we see them covered over with the earth we conclude that all is safe, but if they do not vegetate and come up, they are then pronounced bad seed. We should remember that a very small cavity is sufficient to keep them untouched nearly all around, in which case, under a hot sun, and near the surface, unless they are well pressed after sowing, they are sure to perish. As soon as the plants are well up, they may be thinned out so as to give them two or three inches space; and when the plants will admit they may be thinned out again, giving them fifteen inches space to stand. Those plants that are drawn out may be transplanted. As soon as the grass begins to make its appearance, the tops of the ridges around the plants may be hoed six inches in width. Then, with a single horse-plow, take a furrow from the side of one ridge going up the field, a furrow from the other side coming down, then another furrow from the same side of the first ridge going up, and another from the same side of the other ridge coming down, observing to plow within three or four inches of the plant. This turns a ridge over the original gutter. Then observe to turn these furrows back again to the turnips. In this manner the weeds are nearly, or quite, all destroyed. When the weeds again make their appearance it will be necessary to repeat the same operation with the hoe and plow as before, which may suffice, unless the ground has been uncommonly grassy. Should it be necessary to work it the third time, the application of the hoe may answer. From the above mode of cultivation, the plants or leaves will be so productive as nearly to touch each other in the middle between the ridges. Cobbett states that from the above mode of cultivation, he has raised upward of a thousand bushels from one acre of ground on Long Island, New York, the turnips on an average weighing upward of seven pounds each. Transplanting is a mode said to be preferable, the ground plowed up and made into ridges as above. The plants may be obtained either from those which are thinned out by the first mode of planting, or from seed previously sown in small beds of a rich, light soil, drilled in rows twelve inches apart. They should be thinned out as soon as they are well up, to stand two or three inches apart, in order that the plants may be more thrifty and regular in size. As soon as the plants are large enough, they may be transplanted, giving them the space above mentioned. A moderate season of rain is preferable to too much wet. The mode of planting is as follows: First, the hole is made sufficiently deep — deeper than the root really requires, so that it be not bent at the point, if it can be avoided; then, while one hand holds the plant with its root in the hole, the other hand applies the setting stick to the earth on one side of the hole, the stick being held in such a way as to form a sharp angle with the plant; then pushing the stick down so that its point goes a little deeper than the point of the root, and giving it a little twist, it presses the earth against the point or bottom of the root, and thus all is safe, and the plant is sure to grow. The general and almost universal fault is, that the planter, when he has put the root into the hole, draws the earth up against the upper part of the root or stem; and if he presses pretty well there, he thinks that the planting is well done; but it is the point of the root against which the earth ought to be pressed: for there the fibres are, and if they do not touch the earth closely, the plant will not thrive. The above mode will apply to cabbage and all other plants that are removed. If the ground was plowed or prepared in the fall or winter before, so much the better; the plowing, as before observed, should be very deep, and the ridges well laid up. In this situation it would, by the succession of frosts be shaken and broken fine as powder, by March or April. It should then be turned back, always plowing deep; then, previous to sowing, the manure may be put in the ridges and plowed and sown as first described. As the winters at the North are too severe for the ruta-baga, they are harvested or taken up the last of November, and either put in cellars or hills prepared in such a manner as to keep out the frost. In this climate they would keep in the ground during the winter without injury. The tops, as well as the roots, are excellent food for cattle, hogs, or sheep. By cutting up the roots, and boiling or steaming them, with a little meal added, they are excellent food for hogs.

STRAWBERRIES.

New beds of strawberries may be formed in this climate early in the month of September, made up in beds of four feet and a half or five feet wide, in a good, light soil, neither too moist nor too dry. The most suitable manure for strawberries is composed of rotten leaves or decayed wood, mixed with other rotten vegetable substances scraped from the stable-yard. Walks may be made between the beds, of about two and a half feet wide, sufficient to admit a wheelbarrow, for the purpose of manuring the beds from time to time as may be required. The plants may be procured from the roots that have formed from the runners on old beds, of the growth of the past season, or the year before, which would be preferable, as they would bear more abundantly the next season. Three rows may be set out in each bed; one row on each side, twelve inches from the border, and one row in the middle, so that the plants may have eighteen or twenty inches space from each other both ways: let them be covered two or three inches deep. Should the weather prove dry afterward, they might occasionally be watered a few times of an evening, till they take root. Nothing more need be done, but keeping the soil light and loose between the plants, and free from weeds till frost. After the leaves have become dead or decayed, and before the ground freezes, they may be carefully taken off with the hand close to the crown of the root. The beds may then be covered two or three inches thick with a good coat of manure (half rotted) from the stable or cow-yard, or composed of decayed vegetable mold, as before stated, being careful that it be free from grass-seed of any kind.

5

Early in the spring, before vegetation begins to grow, spread over the beds a slight covering of straw, and set fire to it: this will consume all the decayed leaves, &c., left from last season, and leave the whole neat and clean. The earth may be lightly turned in between the plants, being careful not to injure the roots; then spread on a thin coat of fine manure, well pulverized, raked from the yard, and mixed with ashes, which will warm the ground, and bring on the plants more speedily. After the plants are in a good growing state and begin to blossom, spread on a good covering of fine straw, two inches thick, when the straw is wet and the weather damp, taking care that it be spread on evenly, and that no part of the ground be left bare. This method brings on the fruit earlier, and ripens it finely, and produces a better quality: it likewise keeps the fruit clean, and free from dirt or sand. After this the vines should not be disturbed, until they have done bearing. As soon as the fruit is gone, the runners should occasionally be taken off as they appear, and the beds kept free from weeds during the summer, which may be done by hand as they show themselves. In the fall when the leaves are decayed, the straw may be removed into the stable-yard, and mixed with other manure to rot. If any plants are then missing, they may be replaced with young plants, such as before stated. They should not be set later than the month of September. The beds may then have another coat or dressing, to preserve them from the severity of the winter, as before mentioned. If the above mode is adopted in the culture of the strawberry, they will bear and do well for many years.

Where there are male and female plants, such as

the hautboys are stated to be, it would do well to mix the male plants regularly when setting out, in each row; say one male to every six female plants. A solution prepared as follows may be used with advantage: a pound each of nitrate of potash, glauber salts and sal-soda; and of muriate of amonia a quarter of a pound; dissolved in thirty gallons of rain or river water.

Use this quantity in three applications at intervals of about a week; the first when the green leaves begin to start, and the last just before the plants are in full bloom. Between the applications, when the weather is dry, give them clear, soft water, as the growth of the young leaves is so rapid that, unless watered, the sun will scorch them. Make the application towards evening, with a watering-pot.

OBSERVATIONS ON THE CULTURE OF THE STRAWBERRY, BY A. J. DOWNING.

The strawberry is certainly one of the most valuable and delicious of all the smaller fruits. It is not easily cultivated. It yields an abundant crop in a short time, from a very limited space of ground; and while its pleasant sub-acid flavor is agreeable, and forms one of the most delightful additions to the dessert in summer, it is also extremely wholesome, never, as is the case with most other fruits, undergoing the acetous fermentation. In some diseases it has been highly beneficial, and it is affirmed that Linnæus was cured of the gout by an abundant use of these berries. The strawberry, though a low, herbaceous plant, sends down remarkably strong roots. In good soils these are often found to penetrate to the depth of fifteen inches, or more, in a season. It is neceessary, therefore, to produce a fine bed, that the soil be deep as well as rich: where the sub-soil is not positively bad, the ground is always much improved by trenching (two spades deep) before setting the plants. In doing this, a good coat of manure should be deposited between the two spots. Old garden soils, which have been long cultivated, are astonishingly improved by this practice, the whole becoming renewed by the presence of the fresh soil; and the growth of plants in such mold, when again acted upon by the sun and air, is of course proportionately vigorous. A deep, yellow loam, rather damp than dry, is undoubtedly the preferable soil for this plant: but almost any soil, for so limited a species of culture, may, in the hands of a judicious gardener, be rendered suitable for it. We have seen splendid crops of fruit upon a very stiff, yellow clay, mellowed down by mixing with anthracite coal ashes and manure.

The best season for making new plantations of the strawberry is either in the spring, the latter part of February, or early in March, or directly after the beds have ceased bearing in August. If the latter time is chosen, the plants generally get sufficiently well established to bear a considerable crop the ensuing year. There are various modes in which to plant the beds when formed. Some arrange the plants so as to be kept in hills, others in rows, and others again allow them to cover the whole surface of the bed. We consider the first method preferable, as in that way the ground can be kept cultivated between the plants; the fruit is generally larger and finer, being more exposed to the genial influence of the sun, and the duration of the bed is greater. Three or four rows may be planted in each bed, at a suitable distance apart, and the runners from the rows should be shortened and cut off about three times during the season.

If the plants are not thriving well, a light top-dressing between the rows in autumn will be of great advantage. Burning of the upper surface of the bed in the spring has been highly recommended by some persons; but we have never found it to answer our expectations upon trial. This fruit receives its name from the very ancient custom of placing straw on the beds between the rows of plants, to preserve the berries clean. Clean wheat or rye chaff may be substituted for straw, and it has the very great additional advantage of not only preventing most weeds from growing, by excluding the light, but also, by decomposing with considerable rapidity after the fruit season is past, it contributes much to the enrichment of the surface soil of the bed. Young and strong runners, well rooted, should in all cases be chosen to form the new bed, and not old plants, or those offsets which grow near them.

There is a fact with regard to the strawberry plant little known, the ignorance of which puzzles many a good cultivator. This is the existence of separate fertile and sterile or barren plants in many of the varieties, otherwise plants which produce chiefly male, and others that produce only female flowers. Botanically, the strawberry should produce both stamens and pistils in each flower, and the blossoms should consequently all mature fruit. This is really the case with the alpine, the wood-strawberries, &c., but not entirely so with the large scarlet and pine strawberries. These latter sorts, it is well known, produce the largest and finest fruit, but we very often see whole beds of them in fine flowering condition, almost entirely unproductive. The common parlance in such cases is, that the variety has run out or degenerated; but the idea is a confused and ignorant one, while the healthy aspect of the plants fully proves the vigor of the sort. The truth is, in all strawberries of the foregoing classes, that although each blossom is furnished with stamens and pistils, yet in some plants the pistils are so few that they are scarcely perceived; in others there are scarcely any stamens visible. When the plants bear blossoms furnished with stamens only (or in a large proportion,) they are, of course, barren; when pistils only are produced in abundance, they are fertile. To have a bed planted so as to bear abundantly, about one plant in eight or ten should be staminate, or barren blossoming plants, the others the fertile ones: for, if the latter only be kept, they alone will also be found unproductive. If any person will examine a bed of the Hudson, or any of the large scarlet strawberries, when they are in blossom, he will discover a great number of plants which bear large, showy blossoms filled with fine yellow stamens. These are the barren plants. Here and there, also, he will discover plants bearing much smaller blossoms, filled with the heads of pistils, like a small, green strawberry. The latter are the fertile ones. Now the vigor of the barren plant is so much greater than that of the fertile ones, and their offsets are so much more numerous, that if care be not taken to prevent this, they soon completely overrun and crowd out the fertile or bearing plants: and to this cause only is to be attributed the unproductive state of many beds of the large-fruited strawberries, which are in many instances perhaps entirely devoid of fertile plants.

The proper method, undoubtedly, is to select a few fertile plants of each kind, plant them in a small bed by themselves, and allow them to increase freely by runners; then, on planting, the proper proportion could be made, and kept up by the regular clipping of the runners.

Many of the fine English varieties of strawberries (Wilmot's superb, for instance) are generally found worthless here. This is owing, in some cases, to the ignorance or want of care of those persons who export the varieties, in sending often no fertile plants. In other instances it is equally owing to our negligence here, in not preserving the due proportion of barren and fertile plants. This peculiarity in the blossoms is very little known, or even understood, among scientific cultivators. It was first pointed out to us by our esteemed friend N. Longworth, Esq., of Cincinnati, one of our most distinguished western horticulturists. Its truth we have repeatedly verified, and a slight examination will convince any person of the cause of the numerous worthless, yet thrifty-looking, strawberry beds throughout our gardens. The finest of the large English varieties of this fruit, which we cultivate here, is the Bishop. It is remarkably large, a most abundant bearer, and of superior flavor. Many of the larger-berried sorts, as the Methville Castle, have been hollow and comparatively tasteless, though of uncommon size. This variety, however, appears to us to unite all that can be desired to constitute a strong, fine, and delicious strawberry.

TOMATOES

May be sown any time in the month of April, in a light, rich soil, drilled in rows four feet apart, where they are to remain and grow. They should be sown thinly, and covered one inch deep; and when the plants are well up, they may be thinned out three or four inches apart to give them a good, regular growth. When they are several inches in height, thin them out again to stand three feet apart to remain; then put bushy sticks to them to bear them up, as they spread much and are inclined to run a little. By working them well, and keeping the ground loose and free from weeds, they will bear very abundantly till frost. After the tomatoes are once cultivated, people are not in the habit of saving the seed in the spring, but depend on the volunteer plants coming up from the rotten ones that decay and fall off on the ground in the fall; but to improve and have the genuine sort, it is best to select some of the largest and fairest for seed, and sow every spring. They should be squeezed out, when fully ripe, in water, rinsed well, and dried in the shade for several days. Spread them thinly before they are put away. Bone-dust and common salt is a proper compost to be added to the soil.

PUMPKINS

May do well when planted among corn, where the soil is very strong, and made light and loose; and in order that they may have room, it would be well to plant the corn in drills or rows six feet apart. The corn may be thinned out to stand two or two-and-a-half feet distance between each stalk, which mode is thought best for its growth. Between every other row the pumpkins may be planted, after the second plowing and hoeing, in hills fifteen feet apart, making the hills nearly level with the ground. As the plants will admit, thin them out, so that only one vine may remain to a hill. Hoe and keep them free from weeds as long as practicable without injury to the vines, observing not to hill up the earth around the root. Be sure to take off the first two or three crops when about as large as a goose-egg. When the first crop of pumpkins is gathered, a larger number will occupy their place, which are to be trimmed off. The gathering may be continued so long as time is left for those on the vines to ripen. They are said to produce better when planted apart from other vegetables. The ground should be strong, well pulverized, and made as level as possible, making the hills at least ten or twelve feet apart, keeping the ground loose and free from weeds, as in that mode of cultivation there is less likelihood of injury from drought. They root at every joint, which makes it necessary to have the ground strong and kept loose as they run.

SQUASHES.

All kinds of running squash may be planted about the first of April, and for a succession of crops may be planted till the middle of May, in a similar soil to the pumpkins. Plant free from other vegetables, and observe to take off the first growth when young, as with the pumpkins.

Summer-bush-squash for early use may be planted from the first to the twentieth of April, in a good, warm, light soil, in hills four feet apart. Put several seeds in a hill, but do not leave more than two or three good thrifty plants to grow in each, giving them ten or twelve inches space from each other. As they are cultivated, observe to draw the earth but lightly around the roots.

WINTER, OR LATE RUNNING SQUASHES.

A piece of ground not liable to suffer from drought, free from shade, and sheltered from wind, must be selected. At the proper season plow it three times, or till it is mellow. Dig holes in the earth about eight feet apart, that will contain at least a bushel. Fill each hole about two-thirds full, with good, strong, well-rotted manure, and partly mixed with a good, rotten compost taken from the hog-yard, or hog-pen, adding a pint of dry ashes or lime. Cover the manure slightly with some of the dirt first taken out of the hole, and, after a few days, work it all over thoroughly, and mix with it the best part of the dirt first thrown out, enough to fill up the hole, so as to be a little above the level of the ground. To allow for settling, repeat this working over two or three times in the course of ten or twelve days, and then plant seed from good ripe squashes, which should be done about the last of April, or early in May. The plants will soon spring up and grow vigorously. The yellow-striped bug is the principal enemy to be dreaded. The plants, from the first appearance of the bug, should be examined twice a day, and the pest destroyed. Hoe the ground, and keep it loose and free from weeds, leaving not more than two thrifty plants to a hill. As the vines are liable to be blown about, it would be well to put brush between the hills for the tendrils to lay hold of as they spread. As the ground cannot be worked after the bushes are put down, and the vines spread, it should be kept very clean and free from weeds till then. The few weeds that come up afterwards might be removed, or taken out with the hand.

DIRECTIONS FOR THE CULTIVATION OF WATER-MELONS.

Water-melons, managed as follows, are frequently produced weighing from thirty to forty pounds, as far north as forty-three degrees. If the same pains were taken in the south, they might be raised very large and fine.

Dig holes two feet in diameter, twenty inches deep; fill one foot with rubbish raked from the garden and stable-yard, and unrotted manures; beat down hard, and water it freely; then fill to the top with rich soil; on this spread an inch of fine compost, or well-rotted manure, compact, but not hard. Plant the seed from the fifteenth of April to the first of May, ten or fifteen to a hill, to allow for accidents, a little below the surface of the compost. Brush over the hill with the hand so as to fill the holes made by the fingers; then cover the hill with an inch of clear sand. Should the weather be dry, water them well two or three evenings. The hills may be made twelve feet apart, and when the plants are well up they may be thinned out so as to leave five or six good, thrifty plants: and when the plants have got six leaves, thin out again, so that only two may remain to grow, and give the two plants ten or twelve inches space. If the season be dry, dig down by the side of the hills nearly as deep as the bottom of the holes, and put in a bucket or two of water, filling the hole after the water is absorbed. As soon as the yellow bug is gone, take away the sand, and supply its place with soil. This is all that can be done in the hill. When the plant has six leaves take off the center shoot with the point of a sharp penknife, and when the lateral shoots are six inches long take off all but three. When these begin to fall to the ground, secure them down with cross-sticks; and as they advance, spade up the ground a foot deep in advance of the vines. Once in every three or four feet, put a shovel-full of soil on the leaf-joint of the vine, not covering up the leaf, and press it down gently with the foot on both sides of the leaf. If this is kept moist, it will take root—the ends of the vines to be kept to the ground by cross-sticks. Let the vines spread from the hills regularly so as to cover the whole ground. If the side branches of the main vines are inclined to head up, and not to keep to the ground, take them off, say a foot, from the main vine. All pruning should be done in the middle of the day, when the sun shines. Let no melon grow nearer the root than four or five feet, and then only one on a lateral branch, three to a plant. Let the vine run on as far as it will, keeping it to the ground. Permit no melon to grow that is deformed, and pull off no male blossoms.

When the melon has nearly attained to its size, others may be permitted to grow on the same vine, and a second crop raised. The vines might be made to grow from twenty to thirty feet long. Great care should be taken that they are not moved or trod upon.

The sand is put on the hills as a preventive against the yellow bug; but pumpkin or squash seed may be planted near the hills for the bugs to light on, taking care to pull them up as soon as the bugs are gone. Common salt, bone dust, or superphosphate of lime, guano, ashes, and animal manures, are also good for water-melons.

TO DRIVE BUGS FROM VINES.

The ravages of the yellow-striped bugs on cucumbers and melon-vines, may be effectually prevented by sifting charcoal-dust over the plants. If repeated two or three times, the plants will be entirely free from annoyance. There is in charcoal some property so obnoxious to these troublesome insects, that they fly from it the instant it is applied.

HINT TO FARMERS.

It is said that the spirits of turpentine is a deadly enemy to all the insect tribes, and consequently will destroy the bug or worm which is found to prey on wheat and other grain. With a watering-pot, finely perforated in the spout, a person may sprinkle a field of ten acres, without using more than two or three gallons. The experiment on a small scale may easily be tried.

TO CORRECT DAMAGED GRAIN.

Musty grain, totally unfit for use, and which can scarcely be ground, may, it is said, be rendered perfectly sweet and sound by simply immersing it in boiling water, and letting it remain until the water becomes cold. The quantity of water must be double that of the grain to be purified. The musty quality rarely penetrates through the husk of the wheat; and in the very worst case it does not extend through the amylaceous matter which lies immediately under the skin. In the hot water all the decayed or rotten grain swims on the surface, so that the remaining wheat is effectually cleansed from all impurities without any material loss. It is afterwards to be dried on a kiln, occasionally stirring it; or it would dry in the hot sun if spread there. It should be effectually dried before it is ground, or there would be danger of its heating, and of the flour becoming musty.

POTATOES,

Planted from the middle of February to the middle of April, are raised with the greatest success in this climate: a later planting seldom turns out well, owing, generally, to the heat and dryness of summer. A light soil, which is neither too dry nor too wet, suits them best. The ground should be well plowed once or twice previous to planting, and if the ground was plowed late in the fall, to have the winter exposure, so much the better, in order that the ground might be made mellow and fine. After preparing the ground for planting, lay off the trenches three feet apart, seven or eight inches deep, and throw in the bottom coarse straw or litter from the stable, one or two inches thick, pressing it down evenly; and on this put a compost of stable and cow-pen manure, tolerably well rotted, to about the same thickness; then cut your potatoes, so that there may be one or two good eyes in each piece, from the middle of the potato, rejecting both ends, or what is called the eye or top and the bottom or root end; then drop them in the trench nine inches apart, and cover them with the earth taken from the drill, three or four inches deep, taking care to have the ridge covered very little above the level of the ground. One good molding will be sufficient, after the potatoes get about six or eight inches in hight.

ANOTHER METHOD OF RAISING POTATOES.

The latter part of February, make trenches about ten or twelve inches deep, by running a plow two or three times in a place, and scraping them out with a hoe. In these trenches put a small quantity of stable or other strong manure, drop the potato, and fill the trenches with half-rotted straw or trash from the woods or barn-yard. Then level the ground, and scatter leaves or other trash, about four or five inches deep all over the surface, which keeps the ground moist, and prevents the weeds and grass from growing. There is no trouble in working them afterwards.

A SUCCESSFUL MODE OF KEEPING SWEET POTATOES.

Dig a square pit in the ground about four feet deep, about the size you wish your house to be. Log it upon the inside until the logs are four or five feet above the surface of the earth. Draw the dirt well around the log frame. In the earth, on the inside of the first frame, build another frame of logs, leaving a space of one foot between the two. Fill the space between them with sand or dry earth. Upon the top of the frame lay a plank floor, the upper part of the floor to be covered with earth about four inches deep. Then a roof, with the gable-end opened at the south, and closed at the north. Have a door in the log frame about two feet square, to the south. After the potatoes are dug, they must be protected from the sides and bottom by dry pine leaves. The door must be kept open in warm, dry days, and closed in cold, damp weather, and always at night.

A floor of poles should be made to the potatoe house.

ANOTHER.

Open a hole or bed about a foot deep, in high, dry land (deeper would be better); put the potatoes in a conical form, and cover with fine straw and corn stalks; or stalks alone, at first, and then with earth from eight to twelve inches deep; covering lightly at first, and increasing the quantity of earth as the cold increases, would probably be better, but more risk is run in covering too lightly than too heavily. The only advantage in putting on stalks, is to keep the earth from mixing with the potatoes, as they keep equally well, or better, to put the earth on without either straw or stalks. A house built of clay, the walls about a foot thick, and covered (under the roof) in the same manner, was found not to preserve potatoes. When a hill is opened, remove the contents to this house during winter; but in spring, say early in May, remove the potatoes to a dry house or lot, for if left in the hill, they sprout or become too moist and soft to be good. The yam rarely fails to keep till new potatoes are dug, but the Spanish can seldom be kept so late. Large hills or banks never keep so well as small ones. About twenty bushels are sufficient. The above plan has proved highly successful after much experience.

PRESERVING IRISH POTATOES

Injurious Effects of their Tops.

When digging your potatoes, spread them out as much as possible upon the ground, in order that each potato may feel the direct influence of the sun and air; and do not dig more than can be got in at night, lest they have to be exposed out twelve or twenty-four hours with nothing over them but a few straggling tops, as a sort of apology for a covering. It is recommended to have them carried into the cellar or bins as soon after they are taken from the hills as they can be conveniently. The bins should also be so constructed that potatoes can be excluded from air and light — in short, so as to keep them in a state similar to that which they are in previously to their being dug; that is, secure from the light and air, with a little moisture and a temperature sufficiently low to keep them from vegetating.

The best plan is to make a bin. Put some sand or turf at the bottom, cut some sods, and line up the ends with them, and when the potatoes are put in, cover them over with sods, and beat them down solid. This keeps them moist and cool, and, no doubt, is an excellent plan. The light has a peculiar action on some potatoes, making them heavy and watery or waxy, and strong or rancid to the taste. It is, perhaps, not always possible to prevent this, when they have suffered from some disease of their tops, or have been disturbed while growing, or have not a suitable soil. As it regards the tops, it is generally the custom to throw them down, and take no further trouble about them. It has been recommended to preserve them when green for fodder; and also not to leave them on the ground, as they form a harbor and breeding-place for insects, which will probably injure the next crop, especially if it be wheat. During the past summer, several crops of wheat that succeeded a potato crop, were injured by some worm or insect. It is better, either to gather them up and burn them, or throw them into the hog-yard, for manure.

ANOTHER MODE OF PRESERVING POTATOES FOR FOOD.

An English paper says that to preserve potatoes in a proper state for food for many years, it is only necessary to scald them, or subject them to a heated oven for a few minutes. By doing this they will never sprout, and the farinaceous substance will keep good for many years, provided the cortical part or skin be entire. They should be well dried after being scalded.

TO IMPROVE THE QUALITY OF THE IRISH POTATO.

A way has been recommended for improving the potato from the seed of its own apple. Gather the apples of the blue potato when fully ripe, and wash out the seed, and dry them. In the spring sow them in drills. They come up very thick, having the appearance of small weeds. In two or three weeks they put out leaves, having the appearance of potatoes; then thin and work them. In the fall you will likely have seed of various shapes and complexions, from which select four or five kinds in the spring, and plant each separately. This is said to improve the potatoes very much in flavor and quantity. Wood-ashes will improve the soil for the potato.

ON THE CULTURE OF THE GRAPE-VINE.

There are few things that afford more pleasure for the same expense of time and trouble, than a good and well managed grape-vine. The following plan for its culture has proved, after many experiments, highly successful:—An Isabella vine, one year old from the layer, having a very good root, was planted in the spring in an ordinary soil, of rather a sandy quality, and a wheel-barrow load of wood-yard manure and old lime-mortar put about the root. As soon as it began to grow, all the buds were rubbed off but one, and that was trained perpendicularly, rubbing off during the season all side-shoots; and when it had reached to the top of a second story balcony, the end was nipped off, thus stopping its further growth. In the spring following, every bud but two at the top of the vine were rubbed off, and those two were trained along the front of the balcony on a large wire stretched along the posts for their support. Every side-bud, during this season, was also rubbed off as at first. Both shoots made about thirty-five feet of growth this season. In the second spring, every joint on the horizontal shoots was permitted to send forth its buds, and to grow unmolested, till the branches had fairly set fruit, generally until they were about eighteen inches long. Then the end of each branch was nipped off, and its further growth prevented. The perpendicular stem was carefully prevented from sending out buds. The whole plant was carefully watched that no more buds might be permitted to grow—each one being rubbed off as soon as it appeared. Thus from about the middle of June, the vine was not permitted to form any new wood. During the season the grapes grew uncommonly well, and were very fine, and every one ripened in good season, as was proved by the numerous company at the Horticultural Society exhibition, who unanimously pronounced them the finest grapes there. The produce of the vine was three hundred and fifteen bunches, all very large, and the grapes of uncommon size. The society awarded to them its first premium for native grapes. Almost everybody, however, doubted whether the plant had not been injured by this excessive bearing of fruit; and many old gardeners considered that it would be killed by it. The writer never doubted on this score. He had only compelled the plant to make fruit, instead of wood to be cut off and thrown away; and has no doubt that if he had been able to get, the season before, a greater length of wood for fruit branches, the plant would have supported a much larger quantity of fruit. On trimming the vine, preparatory to its bearing the third year, there was very little wood to be cut off. Only two buds were left on each branch of last year's growth, and these are now growing, and showing fruit-buds very finely. The vine is not dead, nor does it appear to have been injured in the least by last year's hard work. So far, the experiment is highly successful, and we now feel authorized to recommend this plan to all who love fine fruit. It must be borne in mind that the experiment was made with the Isabella grape; we of course cannot say anything about its applicability to other kinds, from experience; but the same reasoning applies with equal force to all kinds. If the powers of a plant can be turned from the formation of wood to that of making fruit, as we have proved it can be, in the case of the Isabella grape, we do not see any reason why the experiment may not be successful with all kinds of grapes and fruit. One thing we do know, that a plant that bears fruit does not grow as much as one that does not; and we are hence authorized to infer, that the power of the plant may be directed at pleasure, either to the growth of fruit or of wood — that by suppressing the one, you may increase the other, to a very great extent. It may be observed that this vine occupies no room at all in the garden. It grows close in the corner of the house, a single stem ascending fourteen feet to the balcony, when it starts off horizontally as above described, along the balcony. Thus every house in any city that has a yard at all, so that the vine may be set in the earth, may have just such a supply of delicious grapes as the writer of this had last fall.

ANOTHER WAY TO CULTIVATE THE GRAPE-VINE.

Why so little attention, comparatively, is bestowed upon the culture of the grape in this country, where there are so many acres of poor land, of little value in an agricultural point of view, but on which vines would flourish and produce largely, and yield a profitable return, is truly surprising. The mode of culture here suggested offers ample means for procuring an abundant supply of this delicious fruit, as hundreds of pounds might annually be produced upon the surface of walling; for every house in town and country has more or less spare walling, which is deemed of no value, and might be turned into invaluable account in the production of the fruit of the vine. There is not a single point of culture in the whole routine of the management of the vine, the knowledge of which is so important as that which enables the cultivator to discover with accuracy the greatest quantity of fruit he can annually extract from it without checking its growth, or impairing its vital powers; for it is well known, that the generous flavor of grapes, and the vital energies of the vine, are much affected by over-cropping. No vine under three inches in girth ought to be suffered to ripen any fruit, and the great end to be attained is the flavor of the grape that is used for the table, and this is regulated by the circumstances under which they ripen; one of which is, the quantity of grapes suffered to remain and ripen as compared with the strength of the vine. Some vines show more fruit than others, but the power to ripen is nearly equal in all. The warmer the aspect, the greater perfection does the grape attain in our climate, as is already demonstrated in the hot-houses; but it is not warmth alone; shelter is equally necessary. There is no period in the growth of the vine, from the moment it is planted until it attains the greatest extremity of its growth, in which any movement of the wind will not have a greater or less pernicious effect on its well-being; for its perspiration is so great through its large leaves, that a great supply of sap is necessary every moment, through the growing season, to enable it to recruit its loss. Every wind that blows on the foliage of the vine deranges its functions, and retards the growth of the plant and the ripening of its fruit, in proportion to its duration and violence. An aspect due-south is a very good one, but the south-west winds form a drawback to its excellence. The best is east by north. I have seen the black Hamburg attain great perfection in this aspect. The soil most congenial to the growth of the vine is a light, rich, sandy loam. One reason why grapes will not ripen on open walls is, the great depth of mold in which the roots of vines are suffered to run, which supplies them with too great a quantity of moisture. The subsoil should be of dry materials, for it is not mere earth the roots require, but air also. Each root requires a peculiar temperature, and all flourish best in a stony soil.

TO PRUNE GRAPE-VINES TO ADVANTAGE.

In pruning vines, leave some new branches every year, and take away (if too many) some of the old, which may be of great advantage to the tree, and will much increase the quantity of fruit. When training the vine, leave two knots or buds, and cut them off the next time; for usually the two buds yield a bunch of grapes. Vines, thus pruned, bear abundantly, whereas others that have been cut close, to please the eye, yielded little or no fruit.

REMEDY AGAINST MILDEW OF GRAPES.

Take a pint and a half of sulphur, and a lump of the best unslacked lime; put them in a vessel of about seven gallons measurement: let the sulphur be thrown in first, and the lime over it; then pour in a pailful of boiling water; stir it well, and let it stand half an hour: then fill the vessel with cold water, and after stirring well again, allow the whole to settle. After it has become settled, dip out the clear liquid into a barrel, and fill the barrel with cold water, and it is then fit for use. Next proceed with a syringe holding about a pint and a half, and throw the liquid with it on the vines in every direction, so as completely to cover the foliage, fruit, and wood. This should be done when the fruit is just forming and about one-third the size of a pea: it may be continued twice or thrice a week for two or three weeks. The whole process for one or two hundred grape-vines need not occupy more than half an hour.

MANAGEMENT OF FRUIT-TREES.

The following suggestions, as to the use of lime around fruit-trees, are worthy of attention. In the autumn, we laid bare the roots of a number of unthrifty apple, pear, and peach trees, and leaving them exposed during the winter, returned the dirt in the spring, and applied to the roots of each tree about half a bushel of gas-lime. Last year the trees seemed greatly improved, and the pears bore more than three times as much as they did the two previous years; the limbs had to be propped up, and the fruit seemed improved. We treated some old quince-trees in a similar manner with success. Ashes are a good substitute for lime, and ordinary lime would probably do as well as the gas-lime. Exposing the roots of trees occasionally during the winter, it is well known, is very salutary.

I have perfect faith in the beneficial use of calcareous substances applied to the roots of trees, sensible, as has been observed, that "oxygen is the basis of acidity," with which all putrid substances are charged; and it is with this view that Major Reybold, of Delaware, the first of the cultivators of the peach (for he and his sons, and sons-in-law, now number 70,000 peach trees-planted in orchards), is at this time actively engaged in dressing his trees with shell-marl by depositing a quantity at the root of every tree, to be pulverized by the frosts of the ensuing winter. He also cultivates his orchard with the plow, turning a shallow furrow over the whole surface of the land, three times during the summer,—a weighty affair, seeing that one of these orchards contains more than one hundred acres; by these means he conceives that he renovates the land and benefits the health of the trees, which are, indeed, in full vigor, although many of them are very old, and as large as some apple-trees of mature growth. One of the proprietors of a lime quarry, mentioned that lime, which was proved by analysis to yield 96.6 per cent. of carbonate, and not a trace of magnesia, increased the size of the fruit of an apricot-tree three-fold, by digging in around its roots a quantity of lime, adding also to its flavor in an equal degree.

MANAGEMENT OF FRUIT TREES.

In the first place, allow me to say that the disease of the peach-tree called and known as the yellows, is not contagious, and I will hold myself ready to prove, not theoretically or speculatively, but practically, that there is no such thing as a healthy peach-tree being infected by another standing adjacent and having the yellows. I will not say that this or any other disease cannot be inoculated; but if it can, I have not been able to do it in several experiments made for the purpose.

I will endeavor to detail some of my experiments and observations in regard to the yellows, &c., and believe that I can show it to be the result of error in their culture. This farm had upon it, a small apple orchard, the trees standing at distances of thirty-two feet; between the rows of apple-trees, peach-trees were planted, at distances of sixteen feet tree from tree. The peach-trees were in a very unhealthy condition; some of them, being in the last stage of the disease called the yellows, ceased to live after that year; others not so bad, but having the disease in the worst form (every part of the tree being affected), received my care and attention. My first desire was to get rid of the peach-worm, which I readily accomplished by the use of salt and saltpetre around the trunks of the trees, &c., and at the same time I gave to those trees producing good fruit, a top-dressing of manure. Two years after, my orchard was entirely free from the worm, and appeared in a healthy condition, with the loss of only three trees out of about forty that had the yellows.

The orchard being in good health, I resolved to test my then theoretical views; having planted a few trees to supply me with fruit in case these should be destroyed, I went more cheerfully to work, and selected eight trees standing in a row, and had the ground manured for about ten or twelve feet on each side of the row of trees; it was then plowed, and potatoes were planted in every third furrow, this furrow receiving an additional quantity of manure. The balance of the orchard was plowed during the month of September; a part thereof received a dressing of manure, and was plowed in; another part was manured after being plowed, and a third part was left without manure; the whole orchard was sown with wheat, and the following spring with clover. The effect was, that a large majority of the peach-trees showed some symptoms of disease, but more perceptible on those where there was no manure, where the manure was turned under, and where the potatoes were planted. Of the eight trees where the potatoes were planted, I was resolved on saving four of them if possible, for here I thought the greatest amount of injury was done (though I have thought differently on this subject since), yet in this case the injury met my fullest expectation, and the four trees unattended to had the yellows and were about to die, when two friends, both peach-growers, came to see my orchard; these gentlemen, pointing to three of these trees, asked if I could cure them; I told them it might be possible, although they were very far gone; their remark was, that they thought these trees could not be restored to health. The middle one of these three trees, being most diseased, was selected by me to be cured; and if those friends will call and see me in September next, I will promise to give them some perfectly sound fruit, to be gathered from this tree, though the fruit is not of a very good kind. The other two trees died for want of attention, and were cut down this spring. Now this is one instance of which I have ample testimony of this disease being curable, though it is not the first instance of cure with me by very many. The disease was produced by the plow, and the cure by rest, with a top-dressing of stable manure and ashes.

I deem it unnecessary to say anything more about my orchard at present, but beg your indulgence to permit me to ask attention to the effect produced from plowing orchards. A person living within two miles of me, has an apple orchard that was, to within the last three years, a most prolific orchard, but in consequence of some of the trees putting on the appearance of decay, he thought that to manure and plow it would be of service; this he did three years ago, and the orchard producing no fruit the next year, and the trees appearing more unhealthy, he manured and plowed again; but still he has no fruit, and his trees are growing worse instead of better. Another person about seven miles distant, has an apple orchard that he has worked in corn three years ago; one of his people being at my house the year following, I inquired if there was any fruit on the trees: "No: the frost has killed all the apples." I then asked him about trees standing in different parts of the orchard, where I knew they could not plow, and was told these trees were full of fruit, and that the "frost did not hurt them." I desired him to say, the next time he was asked why these trees were full of fruit and the others barren, that they had not been injured with the plow. I could give very many instances of this kind, but my object being to call attention to this matter, I will ask every one to make his own observations and comparisons; let every farmer look into his neighbor's orchard and his own, and see what the effect of plowing is when compared with the unplowed orchard adjacent to that plowed; let him call to recollection the fine orchard planted by his father, that is going into decay, and ask himself the cause, and he will receive more knowledge upon this subject than could be derived from volumes written upon orchards—though I would strongly recommend the perusal of all works written upon the subject of our business; the avocations of life are always promoted by a proper and strict inquiry after truth, and no agent should be neglected to the advancement of so desirable an end.

My system is to work a tree just as I do the corn plant; the one as an annual, the other as a perennial; give the tree all the cultivation it is to have while young, and before a set of organs are wanted for the perdurable formation of fruit; and when the tree puts on the appearance of premature decay, I give it a coat of manure spread upon the surface of the ground: this I apply in the fall of the year, always preferring long to short manure, and when ashes are deemed necessary, I have put them on in the spring.

Shall I say a word here about peach-trees many years ago, which Mr. Downing represents to have grown anywhere in the United States, south of 43° of latitude? Well, at that time there was but little demand for peaches as a market fruit, and they were for the most part converted into pork and brandy. For these purposes, it did not answer at that period of time, to pick them off the trees by hand, but a neat grass lay was considered as indispensable to facilitate their collection, as step-ladders are at the present day. The peaches then were shaken off the trees, and the best selected, either for drying or for the still, and the hogs disposed of the remainder.

There were several reasons why orchards were not destroyed at that time by tillage, and perhaps the most prominent one was that a grain crop in the orchard would prevent or retard the gathering of the peaches, which, by the by, were worth more than any grain crop that could be grown in the orchard; but whenever an old peach-orchard was plowed a few times, a new one had to be planted, or at least such was the case 30 years ago, on some farms, to my certain knowledge. I do not wish to be understood that the peach-tree can be grown at the present time with the same facility it could then, for I have no doubt that the pabulum necessary for the support of this tree has become in a great measure exhausted from the soil, but I presume it can be restored; if so, we must get "the neighbors" to resuscitate their soils and to form a good stock by proper tillage; but when tho trees come into full bearing, we must then feel satisfied with whatever Nature may be pleased to do in the premises, for any stirring of the soil after this period of growth is obtained, has a tendency to bring the orchard into decay, of which I can show hundreds of surviving witnesses.

A careful inquiry will show that the peach-tree began to decline about the close of our last war with

England; grain commanding a very high price at that time, peaches were only considered in a secondary point of view, and orchards that probably had not been disturbed with the plow for 15 or 20 years previous, were then put in wheat, corn, &c. This soon brought the orchards into decay, and in many instances they were not replaced; and when replanted, they have been treated very differently from the original. We must now have a crop of grain, grass, or roots, but in former times such things were not expected from a peach orchard after it began to produce full crops of fruit.

ON THE CULTURE OF THE PEACH-TREE.

Having bestowed much time and attention on the cultivation and preservation of fruit-trees, the following are the results of many experiments. After adopting various modes in rearing the peach-tree, none succeeds so well as the following: In the fall of the year I bury the peach-stones (from which I design to raise trees) in a hole under six or eight inches of earth, to remain there until the following spring, when I take them up, and after cracking the stone carefully, so as not to injure the kernels (most of which will be found swollen and ready to sprout), I then plant them in a trench eight or ten inches apart, where they are suffered to remain until the plant has acquired a growth of three or four inches in hight, when I transplant them to the place designed for my peach-orchard, placing small stones about the plant, to preserve them from being trod upon by the cattle, &c. It is unnecessary to be more explicit on this part of the subject; every farmer is acquainted with the mode of rearing, which is emphatically trifling, compared with the preserving of this valuable and delicious fruit-tree. Few have turned their attention to it, and of the few the smallest number have succeeded: perhaps none have fully in preserving the peach-tree from decay for any length of time. I have, however, prevented the destruction of my trees for several successive seasons, and am entirely convinced of the efficacy of my plan in destroying an insect, which, of all other things, I believe most pernicious to the tree. It is a fact, of which perhaps few farmers are aware, that the peach-tree receives its death by an insect of the fly-kind, which annually deposits its eggs in the bark of the root of the tree, sometimes at or near the surface of the ground, but most generally under the surface. The egg is deposited by making small perforations: these are sometimes numerous, and from the circumstance of a gum issuing out of the wounded parts, there is no doubt that it materially injures the health of the tree. Knowing this to be a fact, and believing the insect just alluded to, to be the primary, if not the sole cause of the failure of our peach orchards, I tried a variety of methods to destroy them, and found the following to have the desired effect: In the fall of the year, when the eggs are deposited, I take, for a grown tree, a handful of tobacco-stems, or what will do equally as well, about half a gallon of wood-ashes; and after baring the roots, lay either of them on and about the trunk, and cover the whole with earth. The amber of the tobacco, and the ley of the ashes, are both fatal to the embryo insect, and will effectually destroy it. For young and healthful trees a much smaller quantity will do, as they are seldom disturbed by the insect, from the circumstance of their roots being less exposed than those of an old tree.

Many farmers, in my opinion, injure the health of peach-trees, and bring on premature decay by pruning. I have tried them with and without pruning, and am decidedly against using the pruning-hook at all. The reasons in favor of this plan are obvious. I suffer the tree to grow as Nature pleases, which it does in the manner best calculated to withstand the shocks of storms, and to bear its fruit without props. In pursuing an opposite plan, by cutting off the first branches that appear, a long body is formed, and the tree ultimately divides in two or three main branches, which, when loaded with fruit, or during high winds, are apt to split asunder, and the death of the tree ensues. It is true I have found it necessary sometimes to prop my trees; but they never attain a great height, and take the shape which is given to them by nature. The load is so equally distributed that the necessary propping is easily done. In addition to what I have already stated, it may not be improper to add, that an intelligent farmer informed me, that merely to keep the earth about the root of the tree in the fall of the year, and removing it again when the winter sets in, would destroy the insect, whose eggs would then be exposed to the severe frost. I have never tried this experiment, but am of opinion that it would have a good effect. From its simplicity it is well worthy a trial.

I prefer ashes, because they are always at hand, besides being a good manure for peach-trees. I have found a sandy soil best, both for a nursery and orchard.

PLANTING APPLE-ORCHARDS.

The following mode of planting an orchard of apple-trees is possessed of many advantages. According to the common mode, the trees are planted fifty feet apart, to give them room to spread to their full extent, and that the ground may be worked between them for their benefit, as well as for the crop produced. The disadvantages arising from this plan are so many, as to have suggested the one now proposed in place of it. The disadvantages attending the usual mode of cultivation are: —

1st. The trees grow up with a straight body, six or seven feet high, before they are suffered to produce their limbs. This large body is soon filled with worms under the bark, which is pecked into holes all around by the small wood-pecker searching after them. These two causes soon bring on the canker, which, in a little time, occasions the decay and death of the trees.

2d. They frequently grow crooked and deformed, which is not only unsightly, but a great injury.

3d. Their bodies and large branches become full of moss, and harbor insects which prey upon them.

4th. The trees planted thus, and especially where the ground is cultivated between them, grow luxuriantly, throw out large branches, and form high trees with great heads: thus exposing them to the fury of the winds, which sometimes break off large branches, and which, whenever it happens, if care is not taken to smooth the wound, and protect it from the air, bring on disease and decay. It also renders the fruit liable to be blown down, to the great loss of the proprietor. They are, besides, more difficult to prune and keep in order. Their fruit is more difficult and expensive to gather, owing to the hight and extent of the head, and they seldom bear more than every other, or every third, year.

By the following mode, all these disadvantages, it is believed, will be avoided. The trees are to be planted at every twenty feet; the second spring after planting, head them down at about three feet from the ground, so as to let four branches arise from the part left, taking care to pare away the part from the highest branch down close, so as to let the growing bark cover the wound as soon as possible. This ought always to be well covered with Forsyth's composition, until the scar is completely overgrown by the new wood. The following spring prune all the four branches, which ought to be trained as regularly as they can be had on all sides of the body, each about a foot long, and suffer each of them to put out two shoots, rubbing off with the finger all beside them. Thus you will have from this time eight branches to form its head, and a body only about two feet long. All these eight branches are to be allowed to grow until the tree comes into bearing, taking care to allow no strong-growing, spongy shoot to grow beyond its fellows, but keeping all of equal growth and size. When the tree comes to bear, four of these branches,—every other one,—are to be headed down, each to its lowest shoot, which is to be trained into the vacancy that has been made by lopping away the parent branch. While these four branches are in the progress of making new wood, the four that have been left are bearing, which they will do plentifully for three, four, or five years, until the new wood has come into a bearing state, which may be known by the fruit-buds which they will show in every part. When these new branches have arrived at this state, then cut out the four old ones that have borne fruit, and are now getting up pretty high, and bearing mostly on their tops. Take care in cutting out these old branches to do it as low as you can, and where their lowest shoot is, however small, or where there is even the appearance of a bud to shoot forth and renew them. These are to be trained in the same manner as before directed for the first that were cut out, until they arrive at the state and size to bear fruit in their turn again, when the last bearing ones once more undergo the same operation, and so on alternately.

Note particularly in pruning, or in cutting away these branches, that it must be always done so near to the shoot or bud that grows to furnish the branch in the place of the one cut away, that the growing wood may cover the wound as soon as possible. In all cases where the knife is used, or any injury done in any way, the part must be smoothed, and the composition applied without delay, at any season. The stems, or bodies of the trees, and the branches, are, once a year at least, to be washed with soft soap and water, which, by encouraging their growth, and preventing moss and insects from harboring therein, is of essential service to them. The advantages of this mode are,

1st. The bodies being so short are easily kept clear and free from insects, and of course from the wounds made by the wood-pecker in searching for them, and thus kept healthy and thriving, and of course highly fruitful.

2d. They cannot but be straight, with as many branches on the one side as the other, by which the sap is regularly dispersed, conducing to the beauty, regularity, and health of the trees.

3d. The trees are thus kept in perpetual youth, health, and fertility, and yield an annual crop.

4th. They are not subject to be broken by the high winds, nor their fruit to be lost by being broken off.

5th. They can never contract moss on either body or branches, which greatly injures the large tree.

6th. Their fruit is easily thinned, and more easily gathered, and at less expense; and lastly, the pleasure arising from an orchard thus growing and thus kept is naturally and properly enhanced by the consideration of its superior profitableness.

Let any one go through the State, or the United States, and I will venture to say, that he will find almost every orchard with the body of the trees drilled in holes, and their branches covered with moss; many of the trees bent and crooked; much old, naked, barren, and even dead wood upon them, and scarcely one that bears every year. To all those whose orchards are in this state, this mode offers the only way to resuscitate and renovate them. Cut down trees that are crooked, wounded, irregular, diseased, or decayed, and train up the best and strongest shoot that will put up from the part left, or from the root, and by managing them as above directed, in a few years a young, healthful orchard will take the place of an old, cankery, decayed, unsightly, and unfruitful one. It is scarcely necessary to add, that the more the ground is stirred between the trees the more they will grow and flourish. The best manure for them is marsh mud; salt marsh, if to be had, but never fresh stable manure. The salt in the mud conduces to the health of the trees, destroys slugs, worms, and insects, and this manure carries no weeds into the orchard.

A comparison of the productiveness and profit of an orchard cultivated in the old way, with one treated in the manner now proposed, will show the superiority of the latter over the former in a strong point of view. An acre will contain only sixteen trees at fifty feet apart, whereas it will contain two hundred at twenty feet; the first only bears every other year. Let us then take them when in full bearing, and see their product for a space of ten years. We will allow each large tree to bear twenty bushels; this will give 16 by 20 = 320 bushels for the acre; and as the trees only bear half the time, consequently in the ten years they will produce sixteen hundred bushels. Allow only five bushels per tree for the small orchard, the hundred trees in the acre will produce five hundred bushels, and as they bear every year, the ten years will give five thousand bushels. If it be said the allowance of five bushels is too much for a small tree, let it be remembered that this tree is always in a healthy and fruitful state; that its bearing being renewed every four or five years, it is always young and lusty, and able to bear a good crop. Let it also be remembered that an average of twenty bushels to the large trees is a great allowance, which, I will venture to say, is never realized. Thus, then, whether we consider the beauty, the regularity, the health, or the vigor of the trees on the plan proposed; their greater fruitfulness, and consequent profit; their perpetual renovation and youth; the ease with which their superabundant fruit is thinned and gathered; their greater exemption from injuries from high winds; we cannot but perceive that the advantages are so many, and so decisive, as to give the plan a marked superiority.

FRUIT TREES.

The new method of raising fruit-trees by planting the scions is a great desideratum in the art of obtaining good fruit. It has many advantages over grafting, because it is more expeditious, and requires no stock or tree. They may be planted where they are required to stand, and the labor for one day will be sufficient to plant out enough for a large orchard. After the scions are obtained, the method of preparing the plant is as follows: Take the scion as for grafting, and at any time after the first of February, and until the buds begin to grow considerably, and dip each end of the shoot in melted pitch, wax, or tallow, and bury it in the ground, the buds uppermost, while the body lies in a horizontal position, and at the depth of two or three inches. We are informed that trees obtained in this way will bear in three or four years from the time of planting. We have no doubt of the practicability of this method of raising fruit.

A gentleman in this vicinity the last season planted about twenty scions of different kinds of pears, which appear to flourish. The composition he used was melted shoemaker's wax.

PLUGGING TREES.

This operation is a very efficient remedy for destroying caterpillars, and other insects, preying upon the limbs of fruit-trees, &c.

It has often been desired to find such a remedy. Our shade-trees are covered every year with disgusting and voracious caterpillars. Year after year, new, troublesome, and costly means are proposed, which are inefficient; while this very easy and cheap way to poison and destroy at once all the insects of any tree is so little known, that our farmers and gardeners appear to be unacquainted with it. It was discovered in France, and I have verified it by the knowledge of it everywhere. This simple operation consists in boring a hole with a large spike gimlet about one-third the diameter of the tree in depth. Fill the hole nearly full with the flour of sulphur, and plug it up by driving in a wooden peg. This does not injure the tree in the least, but the sulphur is decomposed, or carried into the circulation by the sap, and is exhaled by the leaves in a gaseous state, while it poisons and kills all the caterpillars and insects preying upon them.

PEACH-WORM.

A mixture of one ounce saltpetre, and seven ounces salt, applied on the surface of the ground, in contact and around the trunk of a peach-tree, seven years old and upwards, will destroy the worm, prevent the yellows, and add much to the product and quality of the fruit. The orchard also may be sown with the same mixture, at the rate of two bushels to the acre.

THE CANKER-WORM.

Take one gallon of cheap whale oil, one pound flour sulphur, twelve ounces sal ammoniac, and one pound chloride of lime. Let the sal-ammoniac and lime be made fine, so that all parts may mix together. Take some old or cheap woollen cloth (about nine inches wide, and in length according to the size of the tree), and tie it round about the middle so as to encircle the tree, letting the upper part of the cloth hang over like the collar of a coat, so as to form a curve for the millers to run into. The cloth may be dipped in the mixture, or it may be well to spread it on with a paint-brush, and it may be well to renew it once or twice a week till the millers have done flying. This was tried last season, after the worms were fully grown. Being shaken from the trees, they attempted to ascend, and would die in two minutes after they came in contact with the above ingredients.

ANOTHER.

A complete remedy against the ravages of the canker-worm has been discovered: it is simply to encircle the tree at the surface of the ground with Scotch snuff. The writer of this has examined trees thus treated, and found the circle of snuff completely fringed with thousands of dead worms. The trees were all tarred, and where the snuff was used, no worms appeared on the tar, and where the snuff was omitted the insects nearly covered the tar.

COMPOSITION FOR HEALING WOUNDS IN TREES.

Melt a pound of tar with four ounces of tallow, and half an ounce of saltpeter, and stir the whole together. A coat of this composition, applied to a cut or bruise, will prevent its decay, and cause the wound to heal. Before applying it, all the unsound part should be cleared away.

CEMENT FOR GRAFTING.

Two pounds and two ounces of rosin, six ounces of tallow, and ten ounces of beeswax. Melt them together, and turn the mixture into cold water, and let it remain till cool enough to handle; then work it as shoemakers' wax. It will remain on the stock for years. It is not so soft as to run in hot weather, nor so hard as to crack in cold weather.

All of the ingredients for making this cement must be of good quality.

SOAP-SUDS FOR WATERING PLANTS.

Every one who has a garden, should have all tho soap-suds saved to water plants with. It will be found to improve the growth of plants very much.

APPLES.

I have statements, without number, of the value of apples for feeding swine. In one case the gain upon raw apples was eleven pounds' weight in twelve days; and in this case nothing except apples was used. The best form of using them seems to be to boil them with potatoes; and it is recommended to put the apples at the bottom of the kettle, and the potatoes thus become impregnated with their flavor. Many farmers pronounce them equal in value to potatoes for the fattening of swine, milk-cows, and beef-cattle. There is no food more healthful or nutritious for human beings than apples, cooked or raw. The free use of apples and milk in place of tea and coffee would give to the young members of the family vigorous bodies and bright minds, and abate a large item in domestic expenses likewise.

GEOLOGICAL DEFINITIONS.

The primitive earths are four; clay, sand, lime, and magnesia. Clay is called by geologists alumina, or argillaceous earth. Sand is called silex, siliceous earth, or earth of flints. Lime, as it exists in the soil, is commonly called calcareous earth. Each of these earths answers a determinate and specific purpose in the economy and growth of plants, and the perfection of the soil lies in the mixture of the whole.

Basis of the whole: the primitive earths which enter into its composition. Vegetable matter: all vegetable substances in a decaying or rotten state. Animal matter: all animal substances in a putrefying state. Organic matter: a term applied both to animal and vegetable substances in a putrefying state. Vegetable mold: the earthy remains of vegetable substances which have either grown or decayed on the soil, or have been conveyed thither in the progress of cultivation. Loam is a combination of vegetable mold with the primitive earth. Marl is a substance consisting of lime, with a small portion of clay, and sometimes of peat, with a marine sand and animal remains. It is useful as a manure, and distinguished by shell, clay, and stone marl.

CORNSTALK SUGAR—DIRECTIONS FOR CULTIVATING THE CORNSTALKS, AND MAKING SUGAR.

With regard to the culture, it is stated that corn should be planted as broom-corn is commonly planted, very close in the row, probably a stalk every three or four inches. The tillage will be the same as for broom-corn. When the young ears begin to appear, pluck them off carefully, and repeat the gathering as often as necessary, so as to prevent the formation of any grain; because, if grain be allowed to form, it takes all the sugar from the stalk. About the time the corn begins to harden, the making of sugar should begin. It is not necessary to say anything about a proper mill to crush the stalk and separate the juice, because mills of the cheapest kinds only should be employed now, until the business would fully warrant an expensive outlay. It would probably be found that the common cider-mill, with plain cylindrical nuts, would be quite sufficient for the farmer who would raise a fourth or half an acre of sugar-corn for his family, and this quantity would be sufficient for a satisfactory experiment.

When the juice is separated from the stalk, about a tablespoonful of whitewash, made of the best quicklime, and about the consistence of thick cream, should be added to each gallon of the juice, and then the boiling should commence. The scum that rises should be carefully removed; and the juice, if this process has been properly conducted, will be quite clear—

nearly colorless. Then commences the process of evaporation; and when the juice has boiled down in about the proportion of eight gallons to one, the boiling will be completed, and it may be poured into a shallow, tight wooden box to grain.

It has been ascertained, that if the juice be boiled in a deep vessel, like the common cooking vessel, sugar will seldom be obtained; while if it be done in a shallow vessel, so that the juice at the commencement of the boiling shall not be more than three to five inches deep, sugar will be obtained without difficulty. It has been ascertained, also, that the sugar from corn will not grain so readily as that from sugar-cane. And in some instances, it has remained more than a week after the boiling, before the sugar was formed, and yet excellent sugar was made.

It should be particularly remembered, that the juice should be boiled as soon as extracted from the stalk. It becomes acid very soon, and no sugar can be made if the juice be allowed to stand two or three hours before it is boiled. The juice will even spoil in the stalk before it is ground, if the stalk be cut off a few hours before grinding. It is necessary, then, that every part of the process should be done with the greatest dispatch. The stalks should be brought to the mill as soon as cut, and ground immediately. The vessel for boiling ought to be properly filled in an hour, or at most two hours, after grinding; and the process of boiling down should immediately commence, and be continued until completed.

Excellent syrup, superior to the best molasses, will be obtained by observing the above directions, and boiling five gallons of juice down to one gallon.

The juice of the corn-stalk is very rich in sugar, when cultivated in the manner suggested. One gallon of juice will produce nearly 1¼ pounds of sugar.

JAUFFRET'S MODE OF MANUFACTURING MANURE.

The first thing to be done, is to prepare a quantity of saturated water, which is done by having a vat made of any convenient size, which is half filled with water, and into which are thrown weeds, and almost any kind of vegetable matter that will ferment readily, so as to fill it, with the water, three-fourths full. He then adds, to a vat twelve feet long, six feet wide, and six feet deep, ten pounds of quick-lime, and five ounces of sal-ammoniac. Then you may add sink-water, refuse from the kitchen, dead animals, and such like matters. Stir it up occasionally, and if it becomes too offensive in odor, add more unslacked lime to it. The next step is to have another vat, smaller than the other, into which sufficient of the above made liquor is to be put to dissolve, or mix with the following materials, which last prepared water he calls Lessive.

Take 200 lbs. of fecal matter and urine (from privies,) 50 lbs. of chimney-soot, 400 lbs. of gypsum (plaster of Paris,) 60 lbs. of unslacked lime, 20 lbs. of unleached wood-ashes, 1 lb. of sea-salt, 10 ozs. of saltpeter, and 50 lbs. of what he calls leaven of manure. Mix all these with the saturating water till it makes a thick porridge. The leaven of manure is the drainings of a former operation, if there has been one. The above ingredients should be mixed as follows: — Stir the first vat up till it is thick, and then pour a portion of it into the lessive vat; into this throw the lime, then the soot, next the ashes, then the fecal matter; and lastly, the saltpeter. The plaster of Paris is to be thrown in little by little, stirring the mixture to prevent caking. When the whole is well mixed, stir in the leaven.

When the above substances cannot be obtained but at too great expense, Jauffret substitutes other things; for instance:—Instead of fecal matter and urine, take 280 lbs. of horse, cow, or pig dung; for the gypsum, 100 lbs. of baked or burnt earth or clayey loam; for the soot, 100 lbs. sheep manure, and the same weight in mud; for the unleached ashes, 50 lbs. of leached ashes or 2 lbs. of potash; for sea-salt, 100 lbs. of sea-water. If you come short of lessive, make it up with the saturating water, always using the most impure and putrid that you can obtain.

Having got the above materials ready, clear away a spot of ground, and beat it hard, so that water will not soak in readily, and make little pits around this plat into which the liquor which drains from the heap may run. Then take your straw, weeds, &c., or whatever you wish to convert into manure, and put them into a vat of lessive; wet and pack them into a heap, treading them down so as to make them compact. At every layer, of a foot, pour on a quantity of the lessive, and tread it in so that the whole shall be well mixed together. The heap may be six or seven feet high, and when all is packed, spread the bottom of the lessive vat on the top so as to slime it all over, beating and pressing all about so as to make it as snug and compact as possible. At the end of 48 hours a fermentation commences. On the third day the top of the heap is to be opened six inches, and the sediment which was thrown on to the top is turned over, and another drenching is given with the lessive, and again covered up as before. On the seventh day, make holes near each other with a fork, say three feet deep, and another drenching given and again covered up. About the ninth day give it another drenching through holes somewhat deeper. In 12 or 15 days the manure will be fit to spread.

It will at once be perceived that it will not do to work upon this in freezing weather. Our readers will also perceive that the principle of manufacturing manure in this way depends on mixing matters in a putrefying and liquid state, to those which are dry and inert, so as to bring about fermentation among the whole, and reduce them to a soluble state; or, as we before expressed it, using a rotten liquor to assist in the decomposition of vegetable matters.

ON PREPARING SEED-CORN.

Dissolve saltpeter in water, so as to make it very strong. Soak your seed-corn therein, until it becomes swelled; then plant it in the usual way, taking care not to let it be long out of the brine before it is covered. It will produce three times the crop, and ripen sooner than the same sort of corn planted without soaking, on ground of the same quality.

WATERING GARDENS.

It is necessary to water gardens for various purposes; as aliment to plants in a growing state, as support to newly transplanted plants, for keeping under insects, and keeping clean the leaves of vegetables. One general rule must be ever kept in mind during the employment of water in a garden; that is, never to water the top or leaves of a plant when the sun shines upon it. It should be done either in the evening or early in the morning, unless the watering be confined to the roots; in which case, transplanted plants and others may be watered at any time; and if they are shaded from the sun, may also be watered over their tops.

Many kitchen crops are lost, or produce inferior quality, for want of proper attention of this kind. The fulness of succulency, which copious waterings in the evenings would impart to vegetables, would amply repay the trouble.

REMARKS

Perform every operation in the proper season, and in the best manner, completing every part of it as you proceed. Finish one job before beginning another. In quitting work for the day, leave all in an orderly manner, making a temporary finish, and putting the tools carefully away.

Keep your walks and every part of your garden in perfect order. A small garden, well tilled, will be more remunerative than a larger one imperfectly tilled.

COOKERY.

CURING AND COOKING MEATS.

GENERAL DIRECTIONS.

MEAT intended for salting should hang a few days, until its fibres become short and tender; instead of being salted as soon as it comes from the market; though in very hot weather it may be requisite to salt as soon as possible, beginning by wiping dry, taking out the kernels and pipes, and filling the holes with salt.

BEEF AND PORK,

After being examined and wiped, should be sprinkled with water and hung to dry for a few hours before they are rubbed with salt; this cleanses the meat from blood, and improves the delicacy. The salt should be rubbed in evenly; first half the quantity of salt, and after two days the remainder. The meat should be turned every day, kept covered with the pickle, and rubbed daily. If required, the brine will serve for more than one parcel of meat, if it be boiled, skimmed, and used cold.

In salting beef, the brisket and flat ribs should be jointed, so as to let in the salt, which should also be rubbed well into each piece. The meat should then be put down tightly in the salt, — the prime pieces at the bottom and covered with salt; the coarse at the top to be used first.

TO CURE HAMS.

Cover the bottom of the cask with salt, lay on the hams with the smooth or skin side down, sprinkle fine salt, then another layer of hams, and so continue until the cask is full. This ought to be of the larger kind. A cask holding sixty-four gallons is small enough, and it would be better if it held one hundred and thirty gallons. Make a brine in the following proportions: six gallons of water, nine pounds of salt, four pounds of brown sugar, four ounces of saltpeter, one ounce of saleratus. Scald and skim, and, when cold, pour the brine into the cask. The hams should remain in this pickle at least three months.

CURING PORK.

As soon as the hogs are dressed, and cool enough to be cut up, pack the side-pieces in a cask or barrel, with plenty of salt on all sides of each piece: and when the cask is full, immediately roll it to the pump, and pump in water until the water ceases to sink in the vessel. Then lay a flat stone, as large as the vessel will receive, on the top, so as to keep the pork always under the pickle; put it in the cellar, covered so as to exclude the flies and air, and there let it remain until a piece is wanted. Care must be taken to keep the meat under the pickle, otherwise it will rust. Here is the whole secret of making good pickled pork for family use.

Alum or rock salt made fine should be made use of for rubbing and putting down the meat in the cask, and if the pork is bloody it would be better to salt the meat well with fine salt on boards for forty-eight hours to let all the blood drain off, and then pack down as above.

TO CURE BACON—SAID TO BE EQUAL TO THE BURLINGTON METHOD OF CURING HAMS.

First salt the pork well with fine salt, and pack it away on boards, with a slope sufficient to let the brine run off. In this situation it lies eight or ten days, when it is taken up, and each piece wiped dry with a coarse cloth, and to each ham and shoulder is added a heaping teaspoonful of the best crystallized saltpeter, by sprinkling over them, and rubbing it well in with the hand. It is then salted well again, and packed away in tight casks, as it then may be an advantage to retain or preserve all the brine you can: whereas the first brine, I have found from experience, to be of great injury, as it tends to putrescence, and should by no means be re-absorbed by the meat lying in it, after being extracted by the salt, as I conceive it to be that which so easily produces the bugs and skippers in the meat after it has been smoked. The time of putting on the saltpeter is of much more importance than is supposed by those who have not made the trial; for if put on at the first salting, the meat is always dry, hard, and too salt. On giving the meat a second salting, I add to the salt as much brown sugar as will moisten or dampen it, and as much of the common red pepper as will give the salt quite a red appearance. The pods are first dried before a fire, or on a griddle, and then pounded fine in a mortar. The meat then lies about five or six weeks, except farther south, where the climate is more moderate;

these four weeks will answer, except the meat be very large and the weather continue very cold. It is then taken out, and each piece rubbed well with hickory ashes, and hung up to smoke with the hock downward, which prevents its dripping, and thereby retains its juice. The coarse alum salt, made fine, should be made use of at the second salting, as it is much more effectual in preserving the meat sweet and pure. Should there not be sufficient pickle from the last salting to cover the hams and shoulders, a strong brine may be made with alum salt, enough to answer the purpose, by boiling it well—observing to skim it while boiling as long as any scum arises, and the brine should not be put on till cold. It is not very essential to add the saltpeter to the middlings, or to cover them with pickle, as they are easily preserved without, particularly when the ribs or bones are taken out, which should be the case when they are large, say when the hogs are over one hundred pounds in weight. It may be well to let the meat hang one day to dry before a smoke is made, which should be done with hickory or oak chips raked up from the wood-pile; and in order to prevent a blaze or too much heat, it would be well to add or mix a little saw-dust made from the hickory or oak wood, or tanner's bark might do very well to add with the oak chips. After the meat is sufficiently smoked, which might be in the course of four or five weeks, if regularly attended to, it might be taken down and packed away in casks or boxes, with charcoal made fine, covering the meat entirely with it; and in the course of the summer it might be taken out once or twice, and examined, and sunned if necessary. The hams and shoulders might be preserved in a good state during the summer if they were sewed up in good stout linen bags, painted or lined, provided it was done early in the spring, before any flies made their appearance. Middlings might remain hung up in the smoke-house, and keep very well by taking them down two or three times to sun, or by making a smoke occasionally under them on a damp day.

TO CURE HAMS SO AS TO PRESERVE THEM FROM FLIES.

For a score of hams, take about three quarts of salt, one pint of molasses, quarter of a pound of black pepper, and two ounces of saltpeter pulverized; mix well together; lay the hams on a table with the rind downwards; rub the mixture over them with the hand, taking care to apply it to every part where there is no rind; let them lay a week, and rub them over with clear salt, which continue once a week for four or five weeks, according to the size of the hams; they are then ready to smoke; or if you choose, after the mixture is sufficiently struck in, put them into brine for two or three weeks before you smoke them; and when smoked, hang them in a dry place. When a ham is cut for use, hang or lay it where you please, the flies will not touch it. We have practised this method for several years, and have no reason to abandon it.

HAMBOROUGH PICKLE.

The following constitutes the famed Hamborough pickle, which has been found to preserve meat effectually, in hot as well as in cold climates:—

Six pounds of alum-salt, eight ounces of brown sugar, and six ounces of saltpeter. Dissolve these articles by boiling in four gallons of water. In this pickle, when perfectly cold, keep any kind of meat sunk and stopped closely. The pickle will also keep beef from being hard and too salt when boiled. Tongues, veal, or mutton, for smoking, should not remain in the pickle longer than ten days. Beef, or tongues, when taken out of the pickle, for boiling, should be kept twenty-four hours in cold water, and then drained before they are boiled.

TO PRESERVE BEEF TENDER AND SWEET THROUGHOUT THE YEAR.

For one hundred weight of beef, prepare the following: Four quarts of coarse alum-salt, made fine; four pounds of brown sugar, and four ounces of saltpeter. Mix these articles well together; then rub your meat with it, and pack closely in the barrel. Sufficient pickle will soon be made in the cask by this process. By no means use any water, as it will spoil the meat when the weather becomes warm. If, at any time, a scum rise on the barrel, skim it off, and sprinkle into it a little fine salt, which will preserve the pickle.—Some persons, fearing their beef will be injured in warm weather, take out the pickle and boil it. This is wrong, as it will harden the beef, and entirely change its flavor.

TO PRESERVE MEAT FRESH FOR A FEW DAYS.

Put the meat into the water running from a spring. It will sink. Examine it daily; when it begins to rise from the bottom, it must be used. It will be found perfectly sound and tender, and may be boiled or roasted. Meat may be preserved in this manner three or four days in summer-time free from taint.—The outside will appear somewhat whitened, but the flavor is not injured. It would be advisable to have a box or tub with a cover, into and out of which the water shall have free passage, which may be put either inside or outside of the spring-house.

TO RESTORE TAINTED MEAT.

If your meat be tainted, take it out of the pickle; wash it so as to cleanse it of the offensive pickle. Then wash your barrel well, with a solution either of lime or ashes, after which re-pack it, and between every layer of meat put a layer of charcoal until your barrel be full; then make a fresh pickle strong enough to bear an egg, and fill up your barrel. As you re-pack your pieces, it would be well to rub each piece with salt. Let it remain a week or ten days, and the taint will have disappeared, and the meat be restored to its original sweetness.

TO SWEETEN MEAT, FISH, ETC., THAT ARE TAINTED.

When meat, fish, &c., from intense heat or long keeping, are likely to pass into a putrescent state, a simple and pure mode of keeping them sound and healthful is, to put a few pieces of charcoal, each the size of an egg, into the pot wherein the fish or flesh is to be boiled. Among others, an experiment of this kind was tried upon a turbot, which appeared too far gone to be eatable. The cook, as advised, put three or four pieces of charcoal under the strainer, in the fish-kettle, and after boiling the proper time, the turbot came to the table perfectly sweet and clean.

COOKING MEAT.

The preparation of meat for the table is usually performed either by boiling, roasting, or stewing; and much of its excellence as food, or value for the purposes of nutrition, depends upon the manner in which these operations are severally performed.

In boiling meat, particularly that which is salted, if the following particulars are observed, the meat will be properly boiled: the water used is better soft —and the meat after being thoroughly washed should be placed over the fire in cold water, that the whole may be gradually heated, and thus boiled equally. Salted meat should never be boiled fast; it is better to be simmered only, as fast boiling makes such meat hard. Pieces of meat chosen for boiling, should be of the same thickness throughout, or they will be unequally cooked. An essential condition of boiling meat properly, and have it retain a good appearance, is to keep the pot well skimmed, and steadily but gently boiling. The coagulated albuminous matter that rises on the surface in boiling, if not removed, will attach itself to the meat and injure both its appearance and flavor. Good cooks allow thirty minutes slow boiling to every pound of meat, reckoning from the commencement of the boiling. Flesh or fish boiled in an open vessel, will leave the lean or fibrous part more tender, than if the vessel is covered. With the farmer, more meat is cooked by boiling than in any other way, and it is, therefore, important that the best and most economical way should always be chosen.

A large part of the meat used in cities is roasted, and every one is aware how much the character of beef or mutton depends on this operation. With regard to the manner of cooking meat in this way, the taste of no inconsiderable portion of the community appears verging to the Abyssinian standard, and we may soon expect to hear that roasting of beef is entirely dispensed with, and that it is eaten by the ultra-fashionables before it has time to cool after being killed. We have some doubts, however, whether man was destined to feed on raw flesh, and believe that the nutritive effect is much increased, and the mechanical labor of the teeth and stomach much diminished, by a proper system of cooking. The true criterion is, that the meat roasted be tender, and this cannot be done by placing it for a few moments before or over a hot fire, by which the outside is burned and the inside left unchanged or raw. The process must be gradual to be complete, and the more perfectly cooked the meat is, the better and more nutritive it will be, and the easier of digestion.

Stewing is nothing else than boiling by means of a small quantity of water or broth, and continuing the operation for a long time to render the substance tender, the texture loose, to make it more sapid, and to retain or concentrate the most valuable parts of animal or vegetable food. The process of stewing must be conducted with a small quantity of water, the heat steady, but gentle, so as to raise the fluid only to a simmering heat, and covered so as to prevent the escape of the fluid by evaporation. Much of the good quality of the dishes prepared by stewing, is dependent on the management of the fire, for if the heat is too great the softening of the meat will not be as perfect, and water must be frequently added, or it would burn on to the vessel. The kinds of meat most suitable for stewing, or which are the most improved by the process, are those that abound in fibrin or lean, and which are frequently too dry or tough for roasting. In stewing, those portions of meat that cannot be eaten roasted, and are rarely boiled, as the hard, muscular or tendinous parts,—the hocks of beef, for instance, — are converted into a rich, gelatinous nutritive food, of the most savory kind, and can be served up with proper vegetables, or used as gravy or soup. In stewing, the great danger is burning the meat by allowing the water to evaporate. This guarded against, stewed meats are excellent.

FRYING PORK.

Take one fresh egg, beat it, add half a gill of sour milk, and a sufficient quantity of flour to make a batter; freshen and fry the pork as usual, then dip the pieces in the batter, which will of course adhere; replace them in the fat, and after a little more frying, a light and delicate cake will enclose the meat, and thus constitute a dish for a middling-sized family, which will tempt the palate of the most fastidious.

TO GLAZE A COLD HAM.

With a brush or quill-feather, go all over the ham with beaten yolk of egg. Then cover it thickly with pounded cracker, made as fine as flour, or with grated crumbs of stale bread. Lastly, go over it with thick cream. Put it to brown in the oven or stove. This glazing will be found delicious.

TO BOIL A HAM.

Hams should always be soaked in water previous to boiling, to draw out a portion of the salt and to make them tender. They will soften more easily if soaked in lukewarm water. If it is a new ham, and not very hard or salt, you need not put it in water till the evening before you intend to cook it. An older one will require twenty-four hours' soaking; and one that is very old and hard should be kept in soak two or three days, frequently changing the water, which must be soft. Soak it in a tub, and keep it well covered. When you take it out of the water to prepare it for boiling, scrape and trim it nicely, and pare off all the bad-looking parts. Early in the morning put it into a large pot or kettle with plenty of cold water; place it over a slow fire, that it may heat gradually; it should not come to a boil in less than an hour and a half, or two hours. When it boils, quicken the fire and skim the pot carefully. Then simmer gently four or five hours more, according to the size. A ham weighing fifteen pounds should simmer five hours after it has come to a boil. Keep the pot well skimmed. When it is done, take it up, carefully strip off the skin and reserve it to cover the ham when it is put away cold. Rub the ham all over with some beaten egg, and strew on it fine bread raspings, through the lid of a dredging box. Then place it in an oven to brown and crisp, or on a hot dish set over the pot before the fire. Cut some writing-paper into handsome fringe, and twist it round the shank-bone before you send the ham to the table. Garnish the edge of the dish with little piles or spots of rasped crust of bread. In carving a ham, begin not quite in the center, but a little nearer to the hock. Cut the slices very thin. It is not only a most ungenteel practice to cut ham in thick slices, but it much impairs the flavor.

When you put it away after dinner, skewer on again the skin. This will make it keep better. Ham should always be accompanied by green vegetables, such as asparagus, peas, beans, spinach, cauliflower, broccoli, &c.

BAKED OR ROAST PIG.

Take out the inwards; take off the first joint of the feet; boil both tender and chop them. Make a dressing of bread soaked soft, the water pressed out, and mashed fine; season with pepper, salt, and sage, adding a little butter, and then fill the pig with this stuffing. To prevent blistering, rub a little butter over the pig. Roast or bake it 2½ hours. The oven should contain a little water; and when the meat is done, mix with a little dressing and gravy from the pan, the chopped feet, &c., and use this for a sauce. Expose the pig to the open air two or three minutes before sending it to the table, first rubbing it over with a little butter, to make it crisp.

TO BARBACUE SHOAT.—A SOUTHERN DISH.

Shoat means a fat young hog, weighing about 24 pounds without head or feet. Make several incisions between the ribs of a fore-quarter, and stuff it with rich force-meat. Put it in a pan with a pint of water, salt, pepper, two cloves of garlick, a tumbler of good red wine, and one of mushroom catsup. Bake it, and thicken the gravy with brown flour and butter. To facilitate the carving, joint and cut the ribs before cooking. Lay the ribs up in the dish. Garnish with balls.

TO BROIL HAM.

Ham is better broiled than fried. Slice it thin, and broil on a gridiron. When dished, place a fried egg on each slice. It should be broiled over bright coals, from five to eight minutes, turning it over once.

TO BOIL HAM.

Put it on in cold water, and let it simmer without boiling, unless very moderately, four or five hours. The water should be changed if the ham is very salt; and, before it is carried to the table, take off the rind. Put over it whole pepper or cloves in diamond figures, if you wish to ornament it in a simple way. A ham, if very dry, should be soaked from twelve to twenty-four hours in warm water before using.

TO TOAST HAM.

After boiling it well, take the skin off; cover the top thick with bread-crumbs, and brown it in an oven.

TO STUFF HAM.

Take a ham well smoked and washed, (let the skin remain on,) and make incisions all over the top two inches deep; stuff them full with chopped parsley and some pepper; — to be eaten cold.

SOUSE.

Clean pig's feet and ears thoroughly, and soak them a day in salt and water; boil them tender and split them. To souse them cold, pour boiling vinegar, spiced with mace and pepper-corns, over them. Cloves give the souse a dark color, but improve the taste. If a little salt be added, they will keep good pickled a month or two.

PRESSED HEAD.

Boil the several parts of the entire head, and the feet in the same way as for souse. All must be boiled so perfectly tender as to have the meat easily separate from the bones; and after neatly separated, chop the meat fine while warm, seasoning with salt and pepper, and other spices to taste. Put it in a strong bag, and, placing a weight on it, let it remain till cold, or put it in any convenient dish, placing a plate with a weight on it to press it; cut it in slices, and serve cold with vinegar, or fry it.

SAUSAGES.

Chop fat and lean fresh pork, (a greater proportion of lean,) very fine, season it very highly with pepper, salt, sage, and other sweet herbs if liked. A little saltpeter tends to preserve them. When fresh pork cannot be had, very good sausages may be made of beef.

To make Bologna sausages, take equal weight of veal, pork, and ham, chopped very fine, seasoned high, and boiled till tender in casings, and then fry them after they are dried.

TO MAKE SAUSAGES.

Take three pounds of nice pork, fat and lean together, chop it as fine as possible, season it with a teaspoonful of beaten pepper, two of salt, about three of sage made fine; mix them well together; have the casings very nicely cleaned, and fill them or put the meat down in a pot. Beef will make good sausages.

SAUSAGES.

Twelve pounds of meat, seven pounds of fat from the back of the chine, five spoonsful of salt, six spoonsful of sage, two of thyme, three of pepper; put into casings, and place in large stone jars, and pour warm milk over, until the jars are full.

OXFORD SAUSAGES.

The following is the recipe for making the celebrated Oxford sausages, so popular in England:—Ingredients—one pound and a half of pig-meat without any skin, and a half pound of veal. One pound and a half of beef-suet, the yolks and whites of five eggs; a dessert-spoonful of sifted sage, after being well dried. Pepper and salt to the taste. Chop the meat small, and then pound it together in a marble mortar, till it is short and tender. Chop the suet very fine, and when the eggs are well beaten together, after the white specks are taken out, pour the liquid over the pounded meat and chopped suet, well kneading together with a clean hand, throwing in the sifted sage, and pepper, and salt, during the operation, so as to let them impregnate the whole mass without being predominant in any part of it. Press the whole, when well mixed, into a wide-mouthed jar, and keep it from the air in a cool place. They may be made up into small balls, or put into casings nicely cleaned, when wanted for use. Use very little grease, or lard, in frying them, as they will be almost fat enough to fry of themselves.

TO MAKE FORCE-MEAT BALLS.

Force-meat balls are a great addition to all made-dishes. Made thus: — take three pounds of veal, and a pound of suet, cut fine, and beat in a marble mortar; have a few sweet herbs made fine, a little mace dried and beat fine, and a small nutmeg grated, a little lemon-peel cut very fine, a little pepper and salt, and the yolk of two eggs; mix all these well together, then roll them in little round balls, and some in long balls; roll them in flour, and fry them brown.

RUMP OF BEEF.

This is the most juicy of all the joints of the beef, but is more frequently stewed than roasted, as it is generally too large to serve whole; cut as much from the chump end to roast as will make a nice dish. When boned, and rolled in the form of a fillet of veal, it will require more time to cook.

A SPANISH STEAK.

Take the tender-loin of beef, have onions cut fine, and put into a frying-pan with some boiling butter; when quite soft, draw them to the back part of the pan, and having seasoned well the beef with pepper and salt, put it in the pan, and rather broil than fry it. When done, put the onions over it, and as much boiling water as will make a gravy after stewing.

STEAK WITH VEGETABLES.

Cut the steak about two and a half inches thick, and longer; dredge it with flour, and fry it in butter a fine brown; lay it in a stew-pan, and pour boiling water into the frying-pan; let it boil, and add it to the steak, which is rendered richer by this process. Slice in turnips, carrots, &c.

VEAL MINCED WITH POTATOES.

Chop some cold veal very fine; add to it an equal quantity of cold boiled potatoes chopped fine; also season with pepper and salt to the taste. Add to it veal-gravy or hot water to moisten it, and plenty of butter; dredge a little flour over it, and put it in a stew-pan over a moderate fire; cover it close for half an hour; when thoroughly heated, it is done.

BRISKET OF BEEF STEWED.

Cut the meat into handsome cutlets, put a piece of butter or clean dripping into a frying-pan as soon as it is hot, flour and fry to a light brown; take it out, and if you have no gravy ready, put a pint of boiling water into the frying-pan, boil for a minute, and strain into a basin, while you make some thickening in the following manner: put about an ounce of butter in a stew-pan, as soon as it melts mix with it as much flour as will dry it up. Stir it over the fire for a few minutes, and gradually add to it the gravy you made in the stew-pan; let them simmer together ten minutes; season with pepper, salt, a little mace, and a wine-glass-full of mushroom-catsup or wine; strain it through a tamis on the meat, and stew very gently till the meat is thoroughly warmed. If you have any ready-boiled bacon, cut it in slices, and put it to warm with the meat.

BOILED RUMP-STEAKS WITH ONION GRAVY.

Peel and slice two large onions, put them into a quart stew-pan, with two table-spoonfuls of water; cover the stew-pan close, set it on a slow fire till the water has boiled away, and the onions are a little browned, then add half a pint of good broth, and boil the onions till quite tender; strain the broth from them, chop them very fine, and season with mushroom-catsup, pepper, and salt; put the onion into it, and let it boil gently for five minutes; pour it into a dish and lay it over the steak. If, instead of broth you use good beef gravy, it will be improved. Stewed cucumbers are also a great addition.

BRISKET OF BEEF.

Take all the bones out of eight pounds of brisket of beef, make holes in it about an inch apart, fill first with fat bacon, second with parsley, third with oysters, and so on until all are filled; also add to the above, pepper, nutmeg, and cloves. When completely stuffed, lay it in a pan, dredge it with flour, pour on it half a pint of water, and the same of broth. Bake it three hours, then skim off the fat, put the meat into a dish, strain the gravy over, and garnish with pickles. Any piece of fresh meat may be dressed in this way, or baked before the fire in a Dutch oven, with onions, the meat being frequently rubbed over with oil.

POTTED BEEF.

Rub two pounds of lean beef with salt and saltpeter, and let it lie two days; then dry the meat, season it with black pepper, and put into a small pan with half a pound of butter; cover it with paste and bake slowly.

BEEF A LA DAUBE.

Lard well a round of beef, and put it in a stew-pan; cut it in slices nearly to the bone, have a few slices of bacon placed around and over the beef, with carrots and onions; season with pepper, salt, and thyme; cover the whole with water, and let it stew very slowly from four to six hours, then take out the round and let it cool. To make the jelly, take all the meat from the stew-pan, strain the broth through a sieve, skim the fat from the top very carefully, put it on the fire with a few grains of pepper, and let it simmer slowly. Beat the whites of four eggs in a cup of water, and stir them in; let it remain on the fire simmering fifteen or twenty minutes. Strain the jelly, and when cool, garnish the meat with it. This dish should be prepared the day before it is used.

TOMATO BEEF.

With eight or ten tomatoes, stew slowly three pounds of beef, cut in slices or slips; add salt, a few cloves, and, just at taking up, a little butter. A gill of tomato-catsup and an onion may be added.

FRICANDEAU OF BEEF.

Lard a piece of lean beef with bacon, seasoned with pepper, cloves, mace, and allspice. Put it into a stew-pan, with a pint of broth or beef gravy, a glass of sherry, a bundle of parsley, and sweet-herbs, a clove of garlic, and a shalot or two. When the meat is tender, cover it closely; skim the sauce, strain it and boil till it is reduced to a glaze. Then glaze the larded side, and serve the fricandeau with tomato sauce.

TO PRESERVE FRESH MEAT.

If fresh meat is rolled up in Indian meal, it will keep well for five days in the hottest weather. It should be laid down in pieces, the weight not exceeding three pounds, and each piece should be entirely covered with meal.

TO KEEP FRESH MEAT IN SUMMER.

Put the meat in a stone jar, and cover it with sour milk; and, by changing it once or twice, it will keep a week or longer. Before cooking, wash the milk from the meat, and lay it in soda-water a few minutes, to make it more tender.

HASHED MEAT.

Cut the meat into small pieces, trimming off all the sinews, skin, and gristle. Prepare the sauce to warm with the meat, and simmer gently till thoroughly warm. It should not boil, as the meat is thereby rendered tough and hard. The sauce may be made as follows: one teaspoonful of Harvey sauce, one of tomato sauce, the same quantity of any other sauce; black pepper, cayenne, salt, half a wine-glass of port-wine, and a couple of capsicums cut fine; mix with the remains of the gravy of beef or mutton of the preceding day. If necessary to thicken, add a little flour from the dredger.

A FINE HASH.

Take any cold game or poultry that you have (you may mix several kinds together); some sausages of the best sort will be an improvement. Chop all together and mix with it bread crumbs, chopped onions aud parsley, and the yolks of two or three hard-boiled eggs; put it into a sauce-pan with a proportionate piece of butter rolled in flour, moisten it with broth, gravy, or warm water, and let it stew gently for half an hour. Cold veal or fresh pork may be hashed in the same manner.

SANDWICHES.

Sandwiches are an elegant and convenient luncheon, if nicely prepared. The bread should be neatly cut with a sharp knife; and whatever meat is used must be carefully trimmed from every bit of skin, gristle, &c.

MINCED COLLOPS.

Take beef and mince it very fine, to which add some salt and pepper. Put this in its raw state into small jars, and pour on the top some clarified butter. When intended for use, put the butter into a frying-pan, and slice in some onions and fry them. Add a little water to it, and then put in the minced meat. Stew it well for a few minutes, and serve.

FRICASSEE OF FOWLS.

Skin and cut up the fowls, and soak them two hours in cold water, to make them white. Drain them. Put into a stew-pan a large piece of butter, and a tablespoonful of flour. Stir them together till the butter has melted. Add salt, pepper, a grated nutmeg, and a bunch of sweet-herbs. Pour in half a pint of cream, put in the fowls and let them stew three quarters of an hour. Before you send them to the table, stir in the yolks of three beaten eggs, and the juice of half a lemon. To keep the fricassee white, cover it (while stewing) with a sheet of buttered paper laid over the fowls. The lid of the stew-pan must be kept on tightly.

A LEG OF MUTTON WITH OYSTERS.

Rub a leg of mutton all over with salt, and put it on the spit to roast with a clear fire, basting it with its own gravy. When it is nearly done, take it up and with a sharp knife make incisions all over it, and stuff an oyster into every hole. Then put it again before the fire to finish roasting. Before you serve it up, skim the gravy well, and give it a boil with a glass of red wine.

VENISON.

Venison is said to be more easily digested than any other kind of meat. It is better kept a day or two after it is killed, before using.

TO ROAST VENISON.

Cover the fat parts with paper and a paste, made of flour and water, to prevent them from burning. Roast a haunch of 12 pounds about four hours. Baste it well, and serve with currant-jelly.

VENISON STEAKS.

Cut the steak into pieces the size you prefer, beat well with a steak-beater, then chop it, and fry with nice lard until done. Thicken the gravy, or sauce, with sweet milk, a little flour and butter, adding pepper to the taste. To be served hot.

MOCK VENISON.

Mutton is the best substitute for real venison. Hang up for several days a loin of fat mutton; then bone it, and take off all the kidney fat, and the skin from the upper fat; mix together two ounces of brown sugar, one ounce of pulverized black pepper, and two of allspice. Rub it well into the mutton, and let it remain in this mixture five days, turning and rubbing it daily. When it is to be roasted, wash off the spices. Serve it with made gravy and currant jelly.

CALF'S HEAD.

Take the half of one, with the skin on; put it into a large stew-pan, with a knuckle of ham, and the usual accompaniments of onions, herbs, &c., and let them simmer, in as much water as will cover the whole, till the flesh may be separated from the bone with a spoon; do this, and while hot cut it into as large-sized squares as the pieces will admit of. The trimming and half the liquor may be put by in a tureen; to the remaining part add half a gill of wine, and reduce the whole of that, by quick boiling, till it is half consumed, when it should be poured over the large square pieces, in an earthen vessel, surrounded with mushrooms, white button onions, small pieces of pickled pork, and the tongue in slices. Simmer till the whole is fit to serve up. Some brown force-meat balls are a pretty addition. After this comes from the table, the remains should be cut up in small pieces, and mixed up with the trimmings and liquor; which, (with a little more wine) properly thickened, will make a very good mock-turtle soup for a future occasion.

FRENCH CHICKEN SALAD.

Take a large, cold, boiled fowl, and having removed the skin and fat, cut the flesh from the bones in very small shreds, not more than half an inch long, and mix with it an equal quantity of celery, cut in small pieces. The dressing should not be made until immediately before it goes to table. Have ready half a dozen or more hard-boiled eggs. Cut up the yolks on a plate, and with the back of a wooden spoon mash them to a paste, adding salt, mustard, cayenne, vinegar, and salad oil, to the taste. Mix all together, until it is a smooth paste. Lay the shred chicken in the middle of a flat dish. Then cover it thickly with the dressing, and mix it thoroughly. Garnish the top of the dish with white lettuce, chopped fine, and the whites of the eggs minced.

TO BOIL A DUCK.

Salt it two days. Boil half an hour; fill with wheat-bread, sage, onions, and butter, rubbed together, also, pepper and salt to the taste. Then return the duck to the pot, and boil until done.

TO STEW A DUCK.

Stuff and half roast the duck, then put it into a stew-pan, with a shred onion, black pepper, sage, winter savory, marjorum chopped fine, and about a pint of beef gravy. Simmer about 20 minutes, then skim it and take out the herbs; add a quart of green peas lightly boiled, and simmer half an hour longer; thicken with a little butter and flour, and serve the duck and peas in one dish. Cabbage boiled, shred and fried in butter, may also be stewed with duck instead of the peas.

TO HASH A DUCK.

Fry a chopped onion in a stew-pan with a little butter; thicken it with flour, then put the duck (cut up) into the sauce to warm, season it with pepper, salt, and a little soy or catsup, and the juice of half a lemon, with a little sugar. Serve in a deep dish, with toasted crackers or bread.

SALINI, OR HOT DUCK SALAD.

Cut off the fillets of roasted ducks into proper pieces; sprinkle over allspice and salt. Add a gill of olive oil, and a glass of claret, or the juice of two Seville oranges. Stir it well over the fire, and serve it.

FISH.

In choosing fresh fish, select only those that are thick and firm, with bright scales and stiff fins; the gills a very lively red, and the eyes full and prominent. In the summer as soon as they are brought home, clean and put them in ice, if you have it, until you are ready to cook them, and never attempt to keep fresh fish two days. Mackerel cannot be cooked too soon, as they spoil sooner than other fish.

Oysters in the shell may be kept a week by the following process: cover them with water and wash them clean with a birch broom. Then lay them with the concave part of the shell undermost, sprinkle each of them well with salt and Indian-meal, and fill up the tub with cold water. Repeat this every day; first pouring off the liquid of the day before. The tub must stand all the time in a cool cellar, and be covered well with a blanket, or something of the sort. If carefully attended to, oysters kept in this way will not only live, but fatten. It is customary to eat fish only at the commencement of the dinner. Fish and soup are generally served up alone, before any of the other dishes appear, and with no vegetables but potatoes. In England, and at some of the most fashionable tables in America, bread only is eaten with fish. To this rule, salt cod is an exception.

TO BOIL FRESH SALMON.

Scale and clean the fish, handling it as little as possible, and cut it open no more than is absolutely necessary. Place it on the strainer of a large fish-kettle, and fill it up with cold water. Throw in a handful of salt. Let it boil slowly. The length of time depends on the size and weight of the fish. You may allow a quarter of an hour to each pound; but experience alone can determine the exact time. It must, however, be thoroughly done, as nothing is more unpalatable than fish under-cooked. You may try it with a fork. Skim it well, or the color will be bad.

The minute it is completely boiled, lift up the strainer and rest it across the top of the kettle, that the fish may drain, and then, if you cannot send it to table immediately, cover it with a napkin in several folds, to keep it firm by absorbing the moisture. Send it to table on a hot dish. Garnish with scraped horseradish and curled parsley. Have ready a small tureen of lobster sauce to accompany the salmon. Take what is left after dinner, and put it in a deep dish with a close cover. Having saved some of the water in which the fish was boiled, take a quart of it, and season it with half an ounce of whole pepper, and half an ounce of whole allspice, half a pint of the best vinegar, and a teaspoonful of salt. Boil it, and, when cold, pour it over the fish, and cover it closely again in a cold place, and it will keep a day or two, and may be eaten at breakfast or supper. If much of the salmon has been left, you must proportion a larger quantity of pickle.

SALMON STEAKS.

Split the salmon, and take out the bone as nicely as possible, without mangling the body. Then cut it into fillets or steaks, about an inch thick. Dry them lightly in a cloth, and dredge them with flour. Take care not to squeeze or press them. Have ready some clear bright coals, such as are fit for beef-steaks. Let the gridiron be clean and bright, and rub the bars with chalk to prevent the fish from sticking. Broil the slices thoroughly, turning them with steak tongs. Send them to table hot, wrapped in the folds of a napkin that has been heated. Serve with them anchovy or lobster sauce. Many epicures consider this the best way of cooking salmon.

Another way is to take pieces of white paper and butter them well. Wrap in each a piece of salmon, securing the paper around them with a string or pins. Lay them on a gridiron, and broil them over a clear but moderate fire till thoroughly done. Take off the paper and send the cutlets to table hot, garnished with fried parsley. Serve up with them prawn or lobster sauce.

TO BAKE FRESH SALMON WHOLE.

Having cleaned a small salmon, season it with salt, pepper, and powdered mace, rubbed on it, both outside and in. Skewer it with the tail turned around, and put to the mouth. Lay it on a stand or trivet in a deep dish or pan, and stick it over with bits of butter rolled in flour. Put into the oven, and baste it occasionally, while baking, with its own drippings. Garnish it with horseradish and sprigs of curled parsley, laid alternately round the edge of the dish, and send it to table with lobster-sauce.

SALMON BAKED IN SLICES.

Take out the bone and cut the flesh in slices. Season with cayenne and salt. Melt two ounces of butter, that has been rolled in flour, in half a pint of water, and mix with it two glasses of port-wine, two tablespoonfuls of catsup, and two anchovies. This allowance is for a small quantity of salmon. For a large dish, you must proportion the ingredients accordingly. Let the anchovies remain in the dish till they are dissolved. Then strain it and pour it over the slices of salmon. Tie a sheet of buttered paper over the dish, and put into the oven. You may bake trout or carp in the same way.

TO COOK COD-FISH.

It is a little surprising that many a good housewife is not aware that the dumb or dried cod-fish ought not to be boiled to have them tender. It operates as with an egg, an oyster, or a clam: the more you boil them, the harder they get. Over-night put the fish to soak in cold water. In the morning it may be removed into a kettle of fresh water, made warm, and set by the fire. Half an hour previous to its being dished up, it may be transferred to a kettle of fresh water, and simmered over the fire nearly to a boiling heat, but no higher. This management does not draw out, but revives and enlivens the nutritious substance in them and leaves the flesh tender and delicious.

TO BOIL MACKEREL IN MARINADE.

Take, with some weak broth, two tablespoonfuls of vinegar, a bunch of sweet-herbs, a few small onions, a dozen cloves, and pepper and salt to the taste; boil them together an hour, then boil the fish in this gravy. Take them out when ready; strain the liquor and thicken it; make it green with chopped parsley, and serve with white gravy-sauce and hard-boiled eggs.

TO BOIL FRESH MACKEREL.

They should be carefully cleaned inside and out, then washed in vinegar and water, and left to dry before being put into the kettle. A handful of salt should be put into the water, which should be cold, and only allowed to boil fifteen or twenty minutes. Use parsley and butter-sauce.

TO BOIL STURGEON.

Having cleaned the sturgeon well, boil the desired quantity in as much water as will just cover it, with two or three bits of lemon-peel, some whole pepper, a stick of horseradish, and a pint of vinegar to every half-gallon of water. When done, garnish with fried oysters, sliced lemon, and horseradish. Serve with melted butter or anchovy-sauce.

GARNISHES.

Parsley is the most universal garnish to all kinds of cold meat, poultry, fish, butter, cheese, &c. Horse-radish is the garnish for roast-beef, and for fish in general; for the latter, slices of lemon are sometimes laid alternately with heaps of horse radish.

Slices of lemon for boiled fowl, turkey, fish, roast veal, and calf's head.

Carrot in slices for boiled beef, hot or cold.

Barberries, fresh or preserved, for game.

Red beet-root, sliced, for cold meat, boiled beef, and salt fish.

Fried smelts for turbot.

Fried sausages, or force-meat balls, around turkey and other fowls.

Lobster, coral, and parsley, around boiled fish.

Fennel for mackerel and salmon, either fresh or pickled.

Currant-jelly for game; also for custard or bread-pudding.

Mint, either with or without parsley, for roast lamb, either hot or cold.

Pickled gherkins, capers, or onions, for boiled meat and stews.

SOUPS.

TURTLE-SOUP.

When the turtle is ready for dressing, cut all the meat that is good for baking, and put it aside for that purpose; then take the bones, fins, entrails, heart and liver, and put them on, with a piece of beef and a little salt, to stew. When about half done, season with black pepper, cayenne, mace, cloves, nutmeg, parsley, and onions chopped fine; thicken with drop-dumplings, made by beating together a thick batter of cream, the yolk of eggs, and a little salt and flour.

MOCK-TURTLE-SOUP.

Scald a calf's head with the skin on, and take off the horny part, which cut in two-inch square pieces; clean and dry them well in a cloth, and put them in a stew-pan with four quarts of liquid, made as follows: Take six pounds of beef, a calf's foot, a shank of ham, an onion, a turnip, two carrots, a head of celery, some cloves and whole pepper, a bunch of sweet-herbs, and a little lemon. Put these into eight quarts of water, and stew them gently, until the liquid is reduced one half; then strain off, and put it into the stew-pan with the horny parts of the calf's head; add some marjoram, savory, thyme, parsley chopped fine, with some cloves and mace pounded, a little Cayenne pepper, some green onions, and half a pint of Sherry wine; stew these gently, till the soup is reduced to two quarts; then heat a little broth, mix some flour, smoothing it with the yolks of two eggs, and stir it over a gentle fire until it is nearly boiling

OYSTER-SOUP.

Take a quart of oysters, drain them with a fork from their liquor, wash them in one water to free them from grit; cut, in small pieces, two slices of bacon; strain the oyster-liquor; then put all together, adding some parsley, thyme, and onions; season with pepper and salt; let it boil slowly, and when almost done, add an ounce of butter rolled in flour, and a gill of good cream. It will take thirty minutes to cook.

SOUP-MAIGRE.

Take of veal, beef cut into small pieces, and a scrag of mutton, one pound each; put into a saucepan, with two quarts of water; put into a cloth one ounce of barley, an onion, a small bundle of sweet-herbs, three or four heads of celery, cut small, a little mace and cloves, three turnips pared and halved, a large carrot cut in small pieces, and a nice bunch of lettuce; cover the pot close, and let it stew five hours; then take out the spice and sweet-herbs, and serve soup.

ANOTHER OYSTER-SOUP.

Take two quarts of oysters; drain them; have ready a dozen eggs boiled hard; cut them in pieces, and pound them in a mortar alternately with the oysters. Boil the liquor of the oysters with a head of celery cut small, two grated nutmegs, a teaspoonful of mace, and a teaspoonful of cloves, with two teaspoonsful of salt, and a teaspoonful of whole pepper. When the liquor has boiled, stir in the oysters and pounded eggs, a little at a time. Give it one more boil, and then serve it up. Salt oysters will not do for soup.

BEEF-SOUP.

A piece of beef, with a handful of rice, and just enough water to cover. Stew four hours over a moderate fire. An hour before it is done, add two or three common-sized onions, ten or twelve common potatoes, (and carrots, if desired,) salt to season, and a half tea-spoonful of pepper. Stir up two or three eggs with milk and flour, and drop in with a spoon; but sliced bread broken in the tureen is still better.

BEEF SOUP.

The best soup is made of the lean of fine fresh beef. The proportion is four pounds of meat to a gallon of water. It should boil at least six hours. Mutton soup may be made in the same manner. Put the meat into cold water, with a little salt; set it over a good fire; let it boil slowly, but constantly, and skim it well. When no more fat rises to the top, put in what quantity you please of carrots, turnips, leeks, celery, and parsley, all cut into small pieces; add a few cloves. Grate a large, red carrot, and strew it over the top; and continue to boil it gently, but steadily, till dinner-time. Next to the quantity and quality of the meat, nothing is more necessary to the excellence of soup than to keep the fire moderate, and to see that it is boiling all the time, but not too fast. Have ready in the tureen some toasted bread, cut into small squares; pour the soup over the bread, passing it through a sieve, so as to strain it thoroughly. Some, however, prefer serving it up with all the vegetables in it. The soup will be improved by boiling in it the remains of a piece of cold roast beef.

BEEF-GRAVY SOUP.

Cut slices of lean beef, according to the quantity wanted, which place in a stew-pan upon sliced onions and roots, adding two spoonsful of rich broth. Soak this on a slow fire for half an hour, stirring it well. When it is sufficiently brown, add more broth, well seasoned with sweet-herbs.

A CHEAP RICE AND MEAT SOUP.

Put a pound of rice, and a little pepper, and broth herbs, into two quarts of water, cover them close and simmer very gently; put in a little cinnamon, two pounds of good ox-cheek, and boil the whole till the strength is incorporated into the liquor.

ANOTHER CHEAP SOUP.

Take an ox-cheek, two pecks of potatoes, a quarter of a peck of onions, three-quarters of a pound of salt, and an ounce and a half of pepper—to be boiled in ninety pints of water, on a slow fire, until reduced to sixty. A pint of this soup, with a small piece of meat, is a good meal for a hearty working man: some of every vegetable, with a few herbs, may be added.

HERRING SOUP.

Take eight gallons of water, and mix with five pounds of barley-meal. Boil it to the consistence of a thick jelly; season with salt, pepper, vinegar, sweet-herbs, and add the meat of four red herrings pounded.

VEAL-GRAVY SOUP.

Garnish the bottom of a stew-pan with thin pieces of lard, then a few slices of ham, slices of veal cutlet, sliced onions, carrots, parsnips, celery, a few cloves upon the meat, and a spoonful of broth; soak it on the fire in this manner, till the veal throws out its juice; then put it on a stronger fire, till the meat catches to the bottom of the pan, and is brought to a proper color; then add a sufficient quantity of light broth, some herbs, and simmer till done.

HODGE-PODGE SOUP.

Take either brisket of beef, mutton, steaks, whole pigeons, rabbits cut in quarters, veal or poultry, and boil some time over a slow fire, in water enough to cover it very well. Add some onions, carrots, parsley, parsnips, turnips, green shallots, one clove of garlic, some allspice, thyme, and basil. When done, drain the meat, place it upon a dish, sift and skim the sauce, reduce some of it to a glaze if desired; glaze the meat with it, then add some gravy in the same stew-pan, and broth enough to make sufficient sauce, with pepper and salt; sift it through a sieve, and serve on the meat. If brisket of beef is used, let it be half done before putting in the roots, which should be scalded first, as the broth is made more palatable thereby.

PORTABLE SOUP.

Cut into small pieces three large legs of veal, one of beef, and the lean part of a ham; lay the meat in a large cauldron, with a quarter of a pound of butter at the bottom; four ounces of anchovies, and two ounces of mace. Cut small six heads of clean washed celery, freed from green leaves, and put them into the cauldron with five large carrots cut fine. Cover all close, and set it on a moderate fire. When the gravy begins to draw, keep taking it off until it is all extracted, then cover the meat with water, let it boil gently four hours, then strain it through a hair sieve into a clean pan, till it is reduced to one-third; strain the gravy, drawn from the meat, into a pan, and let it boil gently until it is of a glutinous consistence; season with cayenne, and pour it an inch thick in dishes, and dry in the sun. Put them up in tight boxes.

You can make a good broth, by adding some fresh cakes to boiling water, or it makes nice sauce for fowls.

SOUP, FLEMISH FASHION.

Scald a half-dozen turkey pinions, a quarter of mutton, and a half-pound of pickled pork; put them all together into a pan, with good broth, a bundle of sweet-herbs, a few cloves, pepper, and salt.

MULLAGA-TAWNY SOUP.

Cut four pounds of a breast of veal into pieces about two inches by one; put the trimmings into a stew-pan with two quarts of water; add twelve corns each of black pepper and allspice. When it boils, skim it well, and let it continue to boil an hour and a half, then strain it off while it is boiling. Fry the bits of veal and four onions in butter, to a nice brown; when these are done, put the broth with them, and put on the fire; when it boils, skim it well; let it simmer half an hour, then mix two spoonfuls each of curry and flour, with a little cold water, and a teaspoonful of salt; add these to the soup, and simmer until the veal is quite tender. Or bone a couple of fowls or rabbits, and stew them in the manner directed above for the veal; and you may add a bruised onion, and some mace and ginger, instead of pepper and allspice.

ASPARAGUS SOUP.

Put a small broiled bone, one and a half pints of peas, and water in proportion, a root of celery, a small bunch of sweet-herbs, a large onion, cayenne pepper, and salt to the taste. Boil briskly for five train and pulp; then add a little spinach juice and asparagus boiled, and cut into small pieces. A teaspoonful each of walnut soy and mushroom-catsup answers as well as the bone.

GIBLET SOUP.

Take four pounds of beef, two of scrag of mutton, and two of scrag of veal; boil them in two gallons of water, stew gently until it begins to taste well; then pour it out, and let it stand till cold, and skim off the fat. Take the giblets of two fowls, well prepared, put them to the broth, and simmer till very tender. Take them out and strain the soup through a cloth. Put a piece of butter, rolled in flour, into the stew-pan, with some fine chopped parsley, chivis, a little pennyroyal, and sweet-marjoram. Place the soup over a slow fire; put in the giblets, fried butter, herbs, a little Sherry wine, some salt, and cayenne pepper; when the herbs are tender, send the soup and giblets intermixed to the table. This forms a very savory dish.

A POOR MAN'S SOUP.

Mince a handful of parsley-leaves fine, and strew over a little salt; shred six green onions, and put them with the parsley in a sauce pan; add three tablespoonfuls of oil and vinegar, with some pepper and salt. Pour over it a nice beef broth, and it is ready to serve.

PEA-SOUP.

Take two quarts of dried or split peas the evening before you intend to make the soup, and let them soak in luke-warm water all night. In the morning put the peas in the pot, with three quarts of cold water, a pound of bacon, and a pound of lean, fre beef. Cut up two carrots, two onions, and two heads of celery, and put them in the soup, with a bunch of sweet-herbs and three or four cloves. Boil it slowly five or six hours, till the peas can be no longer distinguished; then strain it, and serve.

GREEN PEA-SOUP.

Make a good beef-soup with the proportion of four pounds of lean beef to a gallon of water. Boil it slowly, and skim it well. In another pot boil two quarts of green peas, with a little salt, and three or four lumps of sugar. When they are quite soft, take them out, drain the water off, and mash them in a colander till all the pulp drips through. Then stir it into the soup, after you have strained it. Prepare some toasted bread, cut in small squares; lay in a tureen, and pour the soup over. When you toast bread for soups, etc., always cut off the crust.

TO MAKE CALF'S HEAD SOUP.

Take a calf's head, part of the liver and lights, boil them in six quarts of water, until you can take the bones out; put it on a dish, season it with pepper, salt, sweet-marjoram, thyme, sage, mace, and cloves; skim the water, if there be any fat on it; then put it all back in the same water that it was boiled in, and let it boil till done. Just before you take it up, put a glass of wine in it, with a little burnt sugar; thicken it with a little butter and flour.

If you wish to make a great deal of soup, add a knuckle of veal, as the head only will not make it rich enough. If you wish to make the dish without soup, boil the head in the same way, and season it in the same manner in the dish, with a little of the water it was boiled in; thicken it a little with butter and flour: put it in the oven till you think it is done.

OKRA SOUP.

The pods are of a proper size when two or three inches long, but may be used while they remain tender; if fit for use, they will snap asunder at the ends, but if they merely bend, they are too old, and must be rejected; for a few of such pods will spoil a dish of soup.

Take one peck, cut them across into very thin slices, not exceeding one-eighth of an inch in thickness, but as much thinner as possible, as the operation is accelerated by their thinness; to this quantity of okra add about one-third of a peck of tomatoes, which are first pealed and cut into pieces. This quantity can be either increased or diminished, as may suit the taste of those for whom it is intended. A coarse piece of beef (a shin is generally made use of) is placed in a digester, with about two and a half gallons of water, and a very small quantity of salt. It is permitted to boil for a few moments, when the scum is taken off, and the okra and tomatoes thrown in.

These are all the ingredients absolutely necessary, and the soup thus made is remarkably fine. We, however, usually add some corn cut off from the tender roasting ears: the grains from three ears will be enough for the above quantity: we sometimes take about half a pint of Lima beans. Both of these improve the soup, but not so much as to make them indispensable; so far from it, that few add them. The most material thing to be attended to is the boiling, and the excellence of the soup depends almost entirely on this being faithfully done: for, if it be not boiled enough, however well the ingredients may have been selected, the soup will be very inferior, and give little idea of the delightful flavor it possesses when properly done. I have already directed that the ingredients be placed in a digester. This is decidedly the best vessel for boiling this, or any other soup in, but should there be no digester, then an earthen pot should be prepared; but on no account make use of an iron one, as it would turn the whole soup of a black color; the proper color being green, colored with the rich yellow of the tomatoes.

The time which is usually occupied in boiling okra soup is five hours. We put it on at 9 A. M., and take it off about 2 P. M., during the whole of which time it is kept boiling briskly; the cook at the same time stirring it frequently, and mashing the different ingredients. By the time it is taken off, it will be reduced to about one half; but as on the operation of the boiling being well and faithfully executed depends its excellence, I will state the criterion by which this is judged of: — the meat separates entirely from the bone, being done to rags, the whole appears as one homogeneous mass, in which none of the ingredients are seen distinct, the objeet of this long boiling being thus to incorporate them. Its consistence should be about that of thick porridge.

PICKLES AND SAUCES.

TO PICKLE OYSTERS.

Put the oysters on the fire, and let them simmer till the gills begin to shrivel, then take them up and wipe them carefully in a towel; strain the liquor, and put it on to boil, with a little salt, whole pepper, and mace; when well boiled, to a quart of liquor add one half-pint of Sherry wine, and the same quantity of good vinegar; the liquor must be nearly cold before it is poured on the oysters.

TO PICKLE WALNUTS.

Scald slightly, and rub off the first skin of one hundred walnuts, before they have a hard shell. This may be easily ascertained by trying them with a pin. Put them in a strong cold brine, put new brine the third and sixth days, and take them out and dry them on the ninth. Take an ounce of each—of long pepper-pods, black pepper, ginger, and allspice, a quarter of an ounce of cloves, some blades of mace, and a table-spoonful of white mustard-seed; bruise the whole together. Put into a jar a layer of walnuts, strew them well over with the mixture, and proceed in the same manner till all are covered; then boil three quarts of good vinegar with sliced horseradish and ginger, pour it hot over, which may be repeated for three or four days, always keeping the pickles closely covered; add at the last boiling a few cloves of garlic, or shalots. In five months, they will be fit for use.

TO PICKLE CUCUMBERS AND GHERKINS.

Select a sufficient quantity of small, though not too young cucumbers. Put them in a stone pot, and pour over them a strong brine; to this add a small bit of alum, to secure the color. Let them stand a week; then exchange the brine for clear water, in which they must remain two or three days. Boil the best northern cider-vinegar, and, when nearly cool, pour it over the cucumbers, having previously turned off the water. Prepared in this manner, with the addition of cloves, allspice, mustard, and cinnamon, boiled in the vinegar, pickles of every kind will keep for a year. In pickling cauliflowers, tomatoes, and other vegetables which easily absorb the vinegar — the spiced vinegar should be added when cold.

ANOTHER.

To each hundred of cucumbers put a pint of salt, and pour on boiling water sufficient to cover the whole; cover them tight to prevent the steam from escaping, and in this condition let them stand for twenty-four hours: they are then to be taken out; and after being wiped perfectly dry, care being taken that the skin is not broken, place them in the jar in which they are to be kept. Boiling vinegar (if spice be used, it should be boiled with the vinegar) is then to be put to them, the jar closed tight; and in a fortnight delicious pickles are produced, as green as when they were on the vines.

TO PICKLE CUCUMBERS, SMALL MELONS, AND BEANS.

After gathering the vegetables above-named, put them in very strong brine, which make scalding hot, and pour again over the cucumbers, &c., every morning, for ten days; afterwards, boil and pour over every two or three weeks. To prepare them for use, soak the salt out in clear water, changing it every day, until they are sufficiently fresh; then put the vegetables in an iron vessel with cold vinegar; let them remain on the fire until they are near boiling; then take the vegetables out of that vinegar; have other cold vinegar in the vessel they are to remain in; add cloves, mace, ginger, allspice, horseradish, and a table-spoonful of olive-oil, mustard-seed, and green pepper pods. One pound of good brown sugar to each gallon of vinegar.

TO PICKLE SOUR-KROUT.

Chop the heads of large cabbages very fine, and strew it in layers in a barrel, with alternately a handful of salt, mixed with a few caraway-seeds, till the barrel is filled. A heavy weight is next to be placed on the mass, and a fermentation soon commences. After this has subsided, the weight is removed, and the barrel is headed for use. This preparation is highly relished by those accustomed to it, when boiled with beef or pork.

TO PICKLE CABBAGE.

Slice the cabbage crosswise; put it on an earthen dish, and sprinkle a handful of salt over it; cover it with another dish, and let it stand twenty-four hours; put it in a colander to drain, and lay it in a jar; take white-wine vinegar enough to cover it, a little cloves, mace, and allspice; put them in whole; boil it up, and put it over, hot or cold, which you like best, and cover it close with a cloth. Then tie it over with leather.

ANOTHER.

Select the best heads of cabbage, quarter them, sprinkle a good deal of salt on them, and let them remain about five days. To a gallon of vinegar, add an ounce each of mace, allspice, and cloves. Pour the vinegar, boiling hot, on the cabbage, and repeat the boiling and turning it on the cabbage several times, at intervals of two or three days, for two weeks.

TO PICKLE HORSERADISH.

Wash and peel your horseradish, then grate it, add vinegar enough to make it of a proper consistency, and sugar to the taste.

TO MAKE MANGOES.

Gather melons when half grown, or smaller. After cutting out a slice large enough to enable you to take out the seeds, &c., put the melons in brine, and scald as above directed. Use for pickles small cucumbers, beans, green tomatoes, small onions, &c. When all have been prepared, for the cold vinegar, open your melons, fill them with the cucumbers, beans, tomatoes, &c. Season with spices, to the taste. Horseradish and mustard are a great addition. When your melon is full, replace the slice you took out, and confine it by taking a few stitches, which you can easily do. Remove when you wish to put it on the table.

CUCUMBERS, BEANS, RADISH PODS, NASTURTIONS, GHERKINS, AND ONIONS.

Put them in strong boiling brine, reboiling and pouring it over the vegetables every three weeks, until you wish to prepare them for use. Then soak out the salt in clear water, changing it frequently. Then pour on them boiling vinegar, spiced with mace, allspice, ginger, cloves, and sugar, half a pint to a gallon of vinegar.

PICKLED BEETS.

Wash the beets, and be careful not to break any of the roots, then boil in plenty of water, about three hours. Take them up without sticking with a fork. After they have cooled sufficiently, cut them up and pour good vinegar over them. Exclude the air, and they will keep well several months. It will improve them to boil the vinegar occasionally, and pour it hot over the beets.

TO PICKLE GHERKINS.

Take five hundred gherkins, and have ready a large earthen pan of spring-water and salt; to every gallon of water add two pounds of salt; mix it well together, and throw in your gherkins; wash them out in two hours, and put them to drain; let them drain very dry, and put them in a jar; take a gallon of good vinegar, and put into a bell-metal kettle, and add half an ounce of cloves and mace, an ounce of allspice, one ounce of white mustard-seed, a stick of horseradish cut into slices, six bay leaves, two or three races of ginger cut fine, a nutmeg cut fine, and a handful of salt; boil it up in the kettle all together, and put it over the gherkins; cover them close down, and let them stand twenty-four hours, then put them in your kettle and simmer over the fire till they are green. Be careful not to let them boil — if you do, it will spoil them; then put them in your jar, and cover them down close till cold; then tie them over with a bladder, and a leather over that; put them in a cold, dry place. Always keep your pickles tied down close, and take them out with a wooden spoon.

TO PICKLE GRAPES.

Take grapes at the full growth, but not ripe; cut them in small bunches, put them in a stone jar, with vine-leaves between every layer of grapes; then take as much spring-water as you think will cover them, put in a pound of bay salt, and as much white salt as will make it bear an egg; dry your bay salt and pound it, it will melt the sooner; put it into a copper or bell-metal kettle, boil it, and skim well as it boils; take all the black scum off, but not the white scum: when it has boiled a quarter of an hour, let it stand to cool and settle; when it is almost cold, pour the clear liquor on the grapes, lay vine-leaves on the top, tie them down close with a linen cloth, cover them over with another, let them be dried between the cloths; then take two quarts of vinegar, one quart of spring-water, and one pound of sugar, let it boil a little while, skim it as it boils, very clean, let it stand till it is quite cold, dry your jar with a cloth, put fresh vine-leaves at the bottom, and between every layer of grapes, and on the top; then pour the clear pickle on the grapes, fill your jar that the pickle may be above the grapes. Tie a thin piece of board in a piece of flannel, lay it on the top of the jar to keep the grapes under the pickle; tie them up with a bladder, and then a leather.

TO PICKLE PEACHES.

Take your peaches when they are at their full growth, just before they begin to turn ripe; be sure they are not bruised; then take spring-water as much as you think will cover them, make it salt enough to bear an egg, then put in your peaches, and lay a thin board over them, to keep them under the water; let them stand three days, and then take them out and wipe them very carefully with a fine soft cloth, and lay them in your glass jar; then take as much good vinegar as will fill the jar; to every gallon put two or three heads of garlic, a good deal of ginger cut fine, half an ounce of cloves, mace, and nutmeg; mix your pickle well together, and pour over your peaches: tie them close with a bladder and leather, and they will be fit for use in three months. You may pickle nectarines and apricots the same way.

TO PICKLE PEACHES.

Select the white solid or clingstone peach. Put them in brine, and let them remain in it as long as you wish. Boil it occasionally, and pour over the fruit. When you wish to prepare the pickles for use, soak out the salt in clear water. Then boil your vinegar, adding spices, and sugar, to the taste.

SWEET PICKLES.

Put peaches in strong brine for twelve hours, wipe them dry; to each gallon of vinegar, add three pounds of light-brown sugar, three table-spoonsful of ginger, three of spice, and one of cloves. Boil the vinegar and pour over the peaches; the next day boil again, and the pickles will be ready for use. Put them up in small jars, that they may not be long exposed to the air after being opened. Seal the jars tightly.

TO PICKLE TOMATOES.

Gather the tomatoes when they are turning to be ripe. Put them in layers in a jar, with garlic, mustard-seed, horseradish, spices as you like, filling up the jar, occasionally putting a little fine salt proportionably to the quantity laid down, and which is intended to preserve the tomatoes. When the jar is full, pour on cold, good cider vinegar till all is covered; then cork up tight.

SPICED TOMATOES.

Pour boiling water over a bushel of tomatoes and skin them; then boil them well, after which add a table-spoonful each of cayenne and black pepper; a tea-spoonful of salt; half an ounce of cloves; one ounce of mace; mix well, and put the tomatoes in jars, and pour a coating of suet over them, and tie buckskin over the tops. Prepared in this way, they will keep a year.

TOMATOES.

Prick the skins of ripe tomatoes; spread them in layers, and on each layer put pounded mace, cloves, and allspice. Pour vinegar over the whole. The vinegar from tomatoes thus prepared, is a very nice sauce.

HIGDION PICKLE.

Equal parts of green tomatoes and cabbage chopped fine; add onions one quarter the quantity of the above; put all together in a jar; sprinkle salt lightly over each layer; let it remain twenty-four hours, then press it in a towel so as to extract all of the juice; put it back in the jar, and cover it with cold vinegar. Let it remain two or three days; drain the vinegar off, and season the mixture. To each gallon put one tablespoonful of ground mustard, one tablespoonful of black pepper, one of spice, and mace. Add four ounces of white mustard-seed; mix it thoroughly; put it back in the jar, and add cold vinegar; exclude the air as much as possible.

ADDS JAR PICKLE.

Pack the vegetables or fruit — such as cabbage, peaches, or any kind of white pickle — in dry salt, and let them remain three or four days; then take them out (leaving the salt sticking on,) and place in the sun till perfectly dry; then wash off the salt with vinegar and water, and freshen them in cold water. Prepare the vinegar by adding to each gallon a quarter of a pound each of black pepper and black mustard-seed, one ounce each of turmeric and mace, three ounces of cinnamon, one tablespoonful of ground mustard, three cloves of garlic, some horse-radish, and a few onions. Place the pickle in this vinegar; make the jar air-tight, and set it in the sun for two or three weeks. This pickle is very nice indeed.

BEAN SALAD.

Take young tender beans, string, and boil them soft; drain the water off, and while hot, put vinegar, salt, pepper, and a small onion sliced fine over them.

MUSTARD FOR THE TABLE.

Mix eight spoonfuls of flour of mustard with two of salt, and nine of water. Mix to a smooth paste; add six spoonfuls more of water, and mix again.

LEMON PICKLE.

Slice six lemons; rub them with salt; lay them in a stone jar, with two ounces each of allspice and white pepper, and one-fourth ounce each of mace, cloves, and cayenne, and two ounces each of horse-radish and mustard-seed. Pour over them two quarts of hot distilled vinegar; and after standing for a few days, strain. Some add garlic or shallots.

SPICED VINEGAR, FOR PICKLES GENERALLY.

Bruise in a mortar two ounces of black pepper, one ounce of ginger, a half ounce of allspice, and one ounce of salt. If a hotter pickle is desired, add a half drachm of cayenne, or a few capsicums. For walnuts, add also one ounce of shallots. Put these into a stone jar, with a quart of vinegar, and cover them with a bladder wetted with the pickle, and over this, a piece of leather. Set the jar on a trivet near the fire for three days, shaking it three times a day, then pour the mixture on the walnuts or other vegetables. For walnuts, it is used hot, but for cabbage, &c., cold; but to save time, it is usual to simmer the vinegar gently with the spices, which is best done in an enameled sauce-pan.

CRESS OR CELERY VINEGAR.

Pour a quart of the best vinegar over an ounce of cress or celery seeds, dried and pounded. Let them steep ten days; shake every day; then strain and bottle in small bottles.

HORSERADISH VINEGAR.

Pour a quart of best vinegar on three ounces of scraped horseradish, one drachm of cayenne, and an ounce of shred eschalot; let it stand a week. This is very cheap, and you have an excellent relish for cold beef, salads, &c. Horseradish is in perfection in November.

GARLIC AND ONION VINEGAR.

Chop two ounces of the root, put it in a bottle, pour over it a quart of the best vinegar, and shake it well every day for ten days; then pour off the clear liquor into half-pint bottles. A few drops of the garlic will flavor a pint of gravy, as it is very powerful.

GREEN MINT VINEGAR.

Fill a wide-mouthed bottle with the leaves; pour wine or vinegar over them, and let them steep ten days; strain, bottle, and cork tightly. Basil vinegar may be made in the same way.

CUCUMBER CATSUP.

Grate the cucumbers, and squeeze or press out the juice. Measure it, and put as much vinegar to the grated cucumbers as you extract juice. Season with pepper and salt. Bottle and cork tightly, and it will keep well for years.

TOMATO CATSUP.

Boil your tomatoes until they are quite soft, then press them through a hair sieve. Measure the pulp of the tomatoes, and to every quart allow a spoonful of salt; boil it an hour after the salt is in. Have ready in equal proportions, a mixture of powdered ginger, nutmeg, and cloves; add to every quart of the liquid a spoonful of the mixed spices, and a tea-spoonful of cayenne. After stirring in the seasoning, boil the catsup several hours, or until it is as thick as you wish it. Strain it carefully into a pitcher, avoiding the sediment of the spices; then while hot, pour it through a flannel bag into clean bottles. Cork them tightly, and seal the corks. Keep it in a dry, cool place: it will be of a fine scarlet color, and keep any length of time.

PEPPER CATSUP.

Take fifty pods of large red bell pepper-seed, and add to them a quart of vinegar. Boil them until you can mash out the pulp through a sieve. Season with cloves, mace, spice, onions, salt, and two spoonfuls of sugar; then boil to the proper consistency.

PEPPER CATSUP AND MEAT DRESSING.

Nearly fill a stone jar with fresh pepper pods; pour on water enough to cover well, and boil until the mass is soft enough to run through a sieve or colander; add enough good vinegar to make it of the consistency of catsup. After you put in the vinegar, boil together fifteen or twenty minutes. Fill small bottles, cork tight, and set away in a cool place. This catsup is very strong and pungent, and a little of it adds a peculiar relish to cold meats, &c.

COMMON SAUCE.

Soak slices of veal, ham, onions, parsnips, two cloves of garlic, two heads of cloves; then add broth, a glass of white wine, and two slices of lemon; simmer over a slow fire, skim well, and sift.

SAUCE PIQUANTE.

Put a bit of butter with two sliced onions, into a stew-pan, with a carrot, a parsnip, a little thyme, basil cloves, two shallots, a clove of garlic, and some parsley; turn the whole over the fire until well colored; then shake in some flour, and moisten it with some broth and a spoonful of vinegar. Let it boil over a slow fire; skim and strain it through a sieve; season with salt and pepper, and use with any dish requiring to be highly seasoned.

SAUCE FOR VEAL.

Take the bones of cold roasted or boiled veal, dredge them well with flour, and put them into a stew-pan, with a pint and a half of broth or water, a small onion, a little grated lemon-peel, half a tea-spoonful of salt, and a little pounded mace. To thicken it, rub a table-spoonful of flour into half an ounce of butter; stir it into the broth, set it on the fire, and let it boil gently for about half an hour; strain through a sieve, and it is ready to put to the veal to warm up, which is to be done by placing the stew-pan by the side of the fire. Squeeze in half a lemon, and cover the bottom of the dish with toasted bread cut into triangles, and garnish with slices of ham.

KITCHENER'S (DR.) SUPERLATIVE SAUCE.

Claret or port wine, and mushroom catsup, a pint of each; half a pint of walnut or other pickle liquor; pounded anchovies, four ounces; fresh lemon-peel, pared very thin, an ounce; peeled and sliced shallots, the same; scraped horseradish, ditto; allspice and black pepper, powdered, half an ounce each; cayenne, one drachm; celery-seed, bruised, the same; all avoirdupoise weight. Put these into a wide-mouthed bottle, stop it close, shake it up every day for a fortnight, and then strain it, and bottle again.

BREAD SAUCE.

Take four ounces of grated stale bread; pour over it sufficient milk to cover it, and let it soak about three quarters of an hour; then add a dozen grains of black pepper, a little salt, and a small piece of butter; put on a little more milk, and give it a boil; eat it with roast wild-fowl or roast pig.

DRAWN BUTTER.

Melt over the fire a quarter of a pound of butter; throw in a large spoonful of flour, and add half a pint of boiling water and a little salt; boil a few minutes, and then put in a tea-spoonful of cold water. If intended as sauce for pudding, stir in a glass of white wine and half a grated nutmeg.

CELERY SAUCE FOR ROASTED OR BOILED FOWLS.

Take a large bunch of celery, wash it clean, cut it fine, and boil it slowly in a little water till it is tender; then add a little beaten mace, some nutmeg, pepper, and salt, thickened with a piece of butter rolled in flour. Then boil it up, and pour it in your dish. You may add half a pint of cream, and a glass of white wine.

TOMATO-SAUCE, NO. I.

Gather your tomatoes when fully ripe; after washing, mash them in a suitable vessel; then place them in a kettle over a moderate fire, and when just warmed, press a colander down upon them, and dip from the colander all the watery juice. After boiling a short time, strain the mass through a wire-sieve, just fine enough to retain the rinds of the fruit; then return it to the kettle, and boil it to the desired consistency. Just before taking it up, add sugar and spices to the taste. Heat the bottles you intend to use, in a steamer to boiling heat, and while they retain this heat, fill them with the sauce in a boiling state; then cork immediately with good corks, and place them where they will cool slowly. Tomatoes thus prepared, will keep good, and retain all their original flavor, until their season comes around again.

TOMATO-SAUCE, NO. II.

Scald and peel your tomatoes. To each pound, allow a pound of brown sugar, and spices to flavor highly, allspice, cloves, mace, ginger, &c. Simmer all together until the tomatoes are done, but do not allow them to break. Take them up, and to every pound of tomatoes allow a pint of strong vinegar. Exclude well from the air, and it will keep for years.

QUEEN'S SAUCE.

Simmer crumbs of bread in good gravy, until it is quite thick; take it off the fire, and add a few sweet-almonds pounded, two hard yolks of eggs, and a breast of fowl roasted, all pounded very fine. Boil a sufficient quantity of bread to your sauce, and sift all together; then add pepper and salt, and warm it without boiling.

FISH-SAUCE.

Take walnuts at the season for pickling; slice them into an earthen pan; between every layer throw a small handful of salt; stir it with a wooden stick every day for a fortnight; strain the liquor through a coarse cloth, and let it stand to settle; pour off the clear, and boil it with a pound of anchovies to each pint; skim it, and let it stand to cool; give it another boil; add one pint of red port, and one of best white vinegar, to each pint of liquor; also, mace, cloves, and nutmeg, of each an eighth of an ounce; some ground mustard, horseradish, and shallot, or a clove of garlic, in each bottle.

CREAM-SAUCE FOR VENISON.

Run the cream over venison just before frothing it, and catch it in a dish; boil it up with the yolks of two eggs, some onions, and a piece of butter rolled in flour and salt. Half a pint of cream is the proportion for two eggs.

SAUCE ITALIENNE.

Put a piece of butter into a stew-pan, with mushrooms, onions, and parsley, all cut fine; turn the whole over the fire for some time, and shake in a little flour; moisten it with a glass of white wine, and as much good broth; add salt, pepper, and a little mace; beat all fine; let it boil half an hour; then skim away the fat, and serve it up. It will be an improvement to add a bunch of sweet-herbs, which should be taken out before the dish is served up.

NONPAREIL SAUCE.

Take a slice of boiled ham, as much breast of roasted fowl, a pickled cucumber, a yolk of a hard-boiled egg, one anchovy, a little parsley, and a head of shallot, chopped very fine; boil it a moment in good catsup, and use it for meat or fish.

SAILOR'S SAUCE.

Chop a fowl's liver with two or three shallots, and a couple of truffles, or mushrooms; simmer them in a spoonful of oil, two or three spoonsful of gravy, a glass of white wine, and a little salt and pepper. Simmer about half an hour, and skim well before using.

VEGETABLES.

COOKING VEGETABLES.

This branch of cookery, though apparently very simple, requires the utmost attention, and no little judgment.

Vegetables should be boiled in soft water. If it cannot be procured soft, a tea-spoonful of carbonate of soda will render it so.

Take care to wash and cleanse all vegetables from dust and other impurities, before cooking; they should be thoroughly cleansed, for which purpose it will be necessary to open the leaves of cabbage, &c.

With regard to the quality of vegetables, the middle-sized are to be preferred to the very large. Green vegetables, such as cabbage, cauliflower, &c., should be cooked fresh, as they are much better, and more wholesome. Strong-scented vegetables, such as onions, leeks, celery, &c., should be kept apart from delicate ones, such as cauliflowers, &c., or the latter will very soon spoil. Succulent vegetables, such as cabbage, and all sorts of greens, are best preserved in a cool, damp, and shady place. Potatoes, turnips, carrots, and similar roots, intended to be stored up, should not be cleaned of adhering soil, till they are to be cooked.

As the action of frost destroys the life of vegetables, and causes them speedily to rot, and as the air also injures them, all roots should be protected by laying them in heaps, burying them in sand or earth, and covering them with straw or something of the kind.

FURTHER DIRECTIONS.

Vegetables, particularly green, in preparing for dressing, require great attention in point of cleanliness. If vegetables for boiling can be gathered perfectly clean, immediately before cooking, they preserve their color much better without washing, but this will seldom be the case, particularly with those purchased of the green-grocer. When they are a little stale, which is generally the case, if not gathered in your own garden, putting them in water a few hours will freshen them. Salt and water should be used for the purpose of bringing out the slugs, or caterpillars, in which summer cauliflower and cabbage abound. Every drop of cold water, if possible, should be shaken out of them before boiling. Green peas, broad beans, and French beans, ought not to be washed. Turnip-greens, if quite clean and fresh, are better not washed; but if otherwise, they must be washed through several waters.

ASPARAGUS, ARTICHOKES, CELERY, &c.

Scrape the stalks of asparagus clean, tie them up with tape, in bundles of twenty-five or thirty each; cut off the ends of the stalks to equal length. If quite fresh, they need not be washed. Artichokes require thorough washing, and should be soaked at least two hours, in water, before cooking. Celery should be well soaked.

SPINACH.

Pick leaf by leaf, wash it in three waters, put a little salt in the boiling water, boil it very quickly, and keep it under the water; seven or eight minutes will be sufficient to boil it; strain it on the back of a sieve, and press it as dry as possible between two plates; spread it on a dish, and score it crossways, in squares of about an inch. It is often served with poached eggs and buttered toast. It is sometimes stewed in the following manner: when it has boiled five minutes, strain and press it, and put it into a stew-pan, the bottom just covered with rich boiling gravy, and a bit of butter, a little pepper, salt, and two spoonsful of cream; stew it five minutes.

GREEN PEAS.

The common method of cooking this delicious vegetable, by boiling in water, is nearly destructive to its flavor, at least so says a lady who has sent us the following method of preparing them for the table, which, after experience, we must add, is a great improvement: Place in the bottom of the sauce-pan, or boiler, several of the outside leaves of lettuce; put the peas and butter in the dish, in the proportion of two ounces of butter to half a peck of peas; cover the pan or boiler close, and place over the fire; in thirty minutes they are ready for the table. They can either be seasoned in the pan or taken out. Water extracts nearly all the delicious quality of the green pea.

TO BAKE BEETS.

Beets, after being washed carefully, may be baked either whole, like sweet potatoes, or in slices, and served up hot with butter, pepper, &c., to the taste. There is a delicious flavor in beets cooked in this way, which is lost when they are boiled.

RICE FAMILY BREAD.

Make one quart of rice flour into a stiff pap, by wetting it with warm water, not so hot as to make it lumpy; when well wet, add boiling water, as much as two or three quarts; stir it continually until it boils, then add one pint of milk; when cool enough to avoid scalding, add half a pint of good yeast, and as much wheat flour as will make it of the proper consistency of bread; put it to rise: when sufficiently risen, it will be necessary to add a little more wheat flour. If baked too soft, the loaves will be hollow.

TURNIP BREAD.

Let the turnips be peeled, and boiled in water till soft and tender; then strongly press out the juice, mix well together, and when dry, beat or pound very fine, and mix with their weight of wheat meal; then season as you do other bread, and knead it up thin, letting the dough remain a little to ferment; make the dough into loaves, and bake it like common bread.

PUMPKIN BREAD.

The pumpkin is first deprived of the rind, and afterward cut up into slices and boiled; when soft enough it is strained in a colander and mashed up very fine. In this state it may be used in pies, or mixed with flour for pudding, cake, &c. If it be intended for bread, you may add a third or half as much whoat wheat flour as pumpkins. The sponge must be first set in the ordinary way with yeast in the flour, and the pumpkin worked in as it begins to rise: use [illegible] pumpkin as will bring the dough to a proper degree of stiffness without water. Care should be taken that the pumpkin is not so hot as to scald the leaven. It requires more baking than bread made entirely of wheat.

CORN BREAD.

Stir up one quart of Indian-meal with milk, add two beaten eggs and a table-spoonful of melted butter, pour the batter into a bake-pan, and bake slowly with coals on the lid and underneath the pan, or hung over the fire. This is a nice process, and upon the baking greatly depends the flavor of the bread. Eaten warm with butter, we have found it the most delicious kind of bread we ever tasted.

LIGHT CORN BREAD.

Stir four pints of meal into three pints of warm water, add one large tea-spoonful of salt, let it rise five or six hours, then stir it up with the hand, and bake it in a brisk oven.

Another method is to make mush, and before it gets cold, stir in half a pint of meal. Let it rise, and bake as the first.

JUDSON'S CORN BREAD.

Add the well-beaten yolks of four eggs to a pint of buttermilk, and briskly stir in a small handful of Indian-meal. Add a spoonful of drawn butter, and stir in, alternately, the reserved whites well beaten, and meal enough to make a smooth batter of moderate consistence. Add a little soda, quickly turning it into buttered tins, and bake in a brisk oven.

sift the flour into a pan, and pour the milk and butter into it, beat the eggs, and pour them in also; lastly the yeast; mix all well together with a knife; flour your paste board, put the lump of dough on it, and knead it very hard. Then cut your dough in small pieces, and knead them into round balls, stick the tops of them with a fork. Lay them in buttered pans and set them to rise. They will probably be light in an hour; when they are quite light, put them in a moderate oven to bake.

BUTTER BISCUIT.

Half a pound of butter, two pounds of flour sifted, half a pint of milk, or cold water, a teaspoonful of salt; cut up the butter in the flour, and put the salt to it, wet it to a stiff dough with the milk, or water; mix it well with a knife, throw some flour on the paste board, take the dough out of the pan, and knead it very well. Roll it out into a large, thick sheet, and beat it very hard on both sides with the rolling-pin; beat it a long time, cut it out with a tin, or cup, into small, round, thick cakes. Beat each cake on both sides, with a rolling-pin, prick them with a fork, put them in buttered pans, and bake them of a light brown, in a slow oven.

GRIDDLE CAKES, NO. I.

Rub three ounces of butter into a pound of flour, with a little salt; moisten it with sweet buttermilk to make it into paste; roll it out, and cut the cakes with the top of your dredging-box, and bake them on a griddle.

GRIDDLE CAKES, NO. II.

Take a pint of thick milk, or a quart of sour; to the thick add a pint of sweet milk, a little salt, a teaspoonful of soda, and flour to make a batter; the thinner the batter, the more tender the cakes will be, if baked well. Half a tea-cup of cream improves them. Butter while hot. For a sauce, take a teacupful of cream, a spoonful of sugar, and half a teaspoonful of ginger.

PANCAKES OF RICE.

Boil half a pound of rice in a small quantity of water, to a jelly; when cold, mix it with a pint of cream, eight eggs, a little salt, and nutmeg; stir in eight ounces of butter, just warmed, and add as much flour as will make the batter thick enough. Fry in lard, using as little as possible.

BATTER CAKES.

Two eggs well beaten, a tea-cup of milk, a pint of flour, one teaspoonful of soda, one teaspoonful of tartaric acid, and salt to your taste. Leave out the tartaric acid until you are ready to bake.

GRIFFIN BATTER CAKE.

Two eggs well beaten; a common-sized tin cup full of flour; a common teacupful of milk; a teaspoonful of soda; a teaspoonful of tartaric acid; salt to your taste. Leave out one of the powders until you are ready to bake; have your oven pretty hot, and grease it just enough (with fresh lard) to keep it from burning. Send the cakes to the table hot.

BUCKWHEAT CAKES.

Put a large spoonful of yeast and a little salt into a quart of buckwheat, in a jar, and make it into a batter with cold water; let it rise well, and bake it on a griddle. It turns sour very quickly, if it be allowed to stand any time after it has risen. They should be buttered, and served up while hot.

ANOTHER.

In lieu of water, mix up your batter with buttermilk; and instead of leaven or yeast, use a little saleratus (about one teaspoonful to a pint of milk), and two or three eggs.

BATTER CAKES.

One pint of cream, one pint of sour milk or buttermilk, four eggs, a teaspoonful of salt, saleratus sufficient to destroy the acidity of the milk, and three pints of sifted flour, or enough to make a stiff batter. Stir the articles well together, and bake in a deep dish. If for griddle cakes, the batter may be made a little thinner, by not adding so much flour. To be eaten hot with butter.

GREEN CORN CAKES.

Take one quart of green corn, rasped from the ear with a coarse grater, two teacupsful of new milk, one teacupful of flour, mix them together, and add two eggs well beaten; season the batter with salt and pepper, and bake upon a griddle. The corn should be in a state most suitable for roasting or boiling. This preparation makes a capital dish.

TO MAKE PANCAKES.

Take a quart of milk, beat in six or eight eggs, leaving half the white out; mix it well till your batter is of a proper thickness. You must observe to mix your flour first with a little milk, then add the rest by degrees; put in two spoonsful of beaten ginger, a glass of brandy, and a little salt; stir all together; make your stew-pan very clean, put in a piece of butter as large as a walnut, then pour in a ladle of batter, which will make a pancake, moving the pan round that the batter may be all over the pan: shake the pan, and when you think the under side done enough, turn it, and when both sides are done, lay it in a dish before the fire.

WASHINGTON CAKE.

This cake derives its name from the fact that it was a great favorite at the table of General Washington; the last two years of his life, it always formed one of the delicacies of his breakfast-table, and is considered one of the standing dishes of a Virginian.

Take two pounds of flour, one quart of milk, with an ounce of butter, heated together; put the milk and butter into the flour when it is about lukewarm; add one gill good yeast, three eggs, a teaspoonful of salt; place it in a pan over-night, and bake it in the morning in a quick oven for three-quarters of an hour.

FLANNEL CAKES.

Two pounds of flour, six eggs well beaten, one wineglass of yeast, a little salt, wet with milk into a thick batter, and set it to rise. Bake them in small pans.

BANNOCKS.

Scald with milk or water one quart of corn meal; when cool, add two spoonsful of yeast, one teaspoonful of salt, one egg, and one quart of flour. Let it rise, and then add half a teaspoonful of soda. Fry in lard.

BREAD FRITTERS.

Boil a quart of milk, with cinnamon and sugar to the taste. When done, stir in a tablespoonful of rose-water, cut some slices of bread into a circular shape, and soak them in milk; then drain them; have ready some yolks of eggs well beaten, into which dip the slices of bread, and fry them in butter. Serve them with powdered sugar.

FRITTERS.

Make them of any of the batters directed for pancakes, by dropping a small quantity in the pan; or make the plainer sort, and slice apples (pared and cored), into the batter, and fry a slice in each fritter. Currants or sliced lemon make an agreeable change. Fritters for company should be served on a folded napkin in the dish. Any kind of ripe fruit, or sweetmeats, may be used instead of apples.

PUFF FRITTERS.

Boil a pint of fresh milk; while it is boiling, stir in quickly a pint of flour; take it off as soon as the flour is all in. After it has cooled, stir in six eggs well beaten; add a little cinnamon, and set it in a warm place four hours. Then have hot lard in a pan, and drop one spoonful of batter for each fritter. Dip your spoon in cold water frequently, to keep the batter from sticking. For sauce, make thin pap of milk and flour; add to it wine, sugar, nutmeg, and a small piece of butter.

OYSTER FRITTERS.

Make a batter of flour, milk, and eggs; flavor with a very little nutmeg; beard the oysters, and put as many as you think proper in each fritter.

WAFFLES.

Beat four eggs, mix flour and milk to make a thick batter, using a quart of flour, a tablespoonful of melted butter, and a teaspoonful of salt. A half-pint of boiled rice improves them.

WAFERS.

Sift half a pound of flour into a pan; make a hole in the middle, and put in three beaten eggs, a tablespoonful of brandy, a tablespoonful of powdered sugar, one of lard, and a very little salt. Mix all together, adding gradually a little milk, till you have a batter the thickness of good cream. Then stir in a tablespoonful of rose-water. Let there be no lumps in the batter. Heat the wafer-iron on both sides in a clear fire, but do not allow it to get red-hot. Then grease the inside with a brush dipped in lard, or a clean rag with butter tied up in it. Then put in the batter, allowing about two tablespoonsful to each wafer. Close the iron, and in baking turn first on one side and then on the other. When done, sprinkle the wafers with powdered sugar, and roll each one up, pressing the edges together while warm. They should be slightly browned, and of an even tint all over.

COMPOSITION CAKE.

Take five teacups of flour, three of sugar, two of butter, one of milk, five eggs, a teaspoonful of soda, a wine-glass of brandy or wine, a pound of raisins, and a nutmeg. Rub the butter and sugar to a cream; add the eggs well beaten, the spice, and half the flour; dissolve the soda in the milk, strain and mix it with the brandy, and stir it into the cake with the balance of the flour. Add the raisins just before the cake is put into the pan, and bake from three quarters to an hour.

PLAIN COMPOSITION CAKE.

Take a pound and three quarters of flour, one and a quarter of sugar, three quarters of butter, a pint of milk, four eggs, and a teaspoonful of soda. Prepare and bake as the preceding.

CIDER CAKE.

One pound and a half of flour, half a pound of sugar, a quarter of a pound of butter, half a pint of cider, one teaspoonful of pearlash; spice to your taste. Bake till it turns easily in the pans, about half an hour.

CONFECTIONERS' POUND CAKE.

Rub to a cream twenty ounces of sugar, and twelve of butter; stir in twelve well-beaten eggs, a pound and a half of sifted flour, and mace and nutmeg to suit the taste.

POUND CAKE, NO. I.

Rub one pound of sugar, and three quarters of butter, to a cream; add the well-beaten yolks of ten eggs, then the whites, and stir in gradually a pound of sifted flour.

POUND CAKE, NO. II.

Take one and a half dozen eggs; their weight of sugar; and of butter and flour each, the weight of a dozen eggs; cream the butter and sugar together; beat the eggs separately; then beat all well together; add a grated nutmeg, and two spoonsful of rose-water; bake slowly at first, adding heat gradually, for the cake to rise; then bake in a moderately quick oven.

POUND CAKE, NO. III.

Take a pound of butter, beat it in an earthen pan with your hand one way till it is like a fine thick cream; then have ready twelve eggs, put half the whites, beat them well, and beat them up with the butter, a pound of flour beat in it, a pound of sugar, a pound of currants, clean washed and picked, and a few caraways. Beat it all well together for an hour with your hands, or a large wooden spoon: butter a pan and put it in, and then bake it an hour in a quick oven.

SPONGE CAKE, NO. I.

One pound of sugar, a half-gill of boiling water, eight eggs, one pound of flour. Pour the water on the sugar, when cool, mix first with the yolks, and then the whites.

SPONGE CAKE, NO. II.

Twelve eggs, a half-pound of flour, one pound of sugar. Beat the whites and yolks of the eggs separately, add next the sugar to the yolks, then the whites; lastly the flour, and stir it in lightly. Bake in a quick oven immediately after adding the juice of a lemon, also the rind grated fine, and a nutmeg.

Sponge cake should not be beaten any after the flour has been added, as it will prevent it from being light.

SPONGE CAKE, NO. III.

Four large eggs, two cups of flour, two cups of sugar, one teaspoonful of soda, and rose-water, and nutmeg to flavor. Beat the eggs separately, then add the sugar to the yolks, next the whites, lastly the flour. Stir in the flour gently, or the cake will not be light. Bake in a moderate oven.

CHEAP SPONGE CAKE.

Four eggs, three cups of sugar, one cup of milk, one teaspoonful of soda, flour enough to make a stiff batter, spices to the taste. Bake in a quick oven.

SPONGE BISCUIT.

Beat ten eggs very thick and smooth, and add gradually a pound of powdered refined sugar; grate the peel of a lemon, and stir it into the mixture. Squeeze in the juice of the lemon, and add two table-spoonsful of rose-water. Beat the mixture very hard; then take half a pound of potato flour (which is best), or else of fine wheat flour, and stir it in very lightly and slowly. It must be baked immediately.

Have ready some small square or oblong cases of thick white paper, with an edge turned up all around, and sewed at the corners. They should be about a finger in length, half a finger in breadth, and an inch and a half in depth. Either butter these paper cases, or sift white sugar all over the inside; then put some of the mixture in each case, but do not fill them to the top; grate loaf-sugar over the top of each, and bake them quickly.

These cakes are much better when baked in paper cases, tins being generally too thick for them; no cake requires greater care in baking. If the oven is not hot enough, both at top and bottom, they will fall and be heavy, and lose their shape.

RICE CAKE.

Take half a pound of rice and wash it well, put it into a pint of cream, or milk, and boil it soft; let it get cold, then stir into it alternately a quarter of a pound of sugar, two ounces of butter, eight eggs, well beaten (having left out the whites of four), and a wine-glass of rose-water, or else the grated peel of a lemon. Mix all well, butter a mold or a deep pan with straight sides, and spread grated bread crumbs all over its inside. Put in the mixture, and bake it three-quarters of an hour. Ground rice is the best for this cake. If any of the cake is left, you may next day cut it into slices, and fry them in butter.

Or, instead of baking the mixture in a large cake, you may put flour on your hands, and roll it into balls. Make a batter of beaten eggs, sugar, and grated bread; dip the balls into it, and fry them in butter.

POTATO CAKE.

Roast in the ashes a dozen small, or six large potatoes. When done, peel them, and put them into a pan with a little salt, and the rind of a lemon grated. Add a quarter of a pound of butter, or half a pint of cream, and a quarter of a pound of sugar. Having mashed the potatoes with this mixture, rub it through a colander, and stir it very hard; then set it away to cool. Beat eight eggs, and stir them gradually into the mixture. Season it with a teaspoonful of mixed spice, and half a glass of rose-water; butter a mold or a deep dish, and spread the inside all over with grated bread; put in the mixture, and bake it for three-quarters of an hour.

FRUIT CAKE.

One pound of sugar rolled, and beaten with a pound of butter; one pound of flour; one pound of currants; half a pound of seeded raisins; a wine-glass of brandy; a grated nutmeg; a little mace; ten eggs, and half a pound of citron; beat the yolks first, and mix in with the other ingredients; then beat the whites as light as possible, and add them. Bake about an hour and a half.

SILVER CAKE.

The whites of six eggs, half a cup of butter, three-fourths of a cup of sweet milk, one cup of sugar, two cups of flour, one teaspoonful of cream of tartar, half a teaspoonful of soda.

ELECTION CAKE.

Four quarts of flour, three-quarters of a pound of butter, four eggs, one pound of sugar, one pound of currants, or raisins, half a pint of good yeast. Moisten it with milk, over-night, in winter; and in warm weather three hours is usually enough for it to rise.

CHEAP AND EXCELLENT CAKE.

Two cups of sugar, two cups of buttermilk, eight cups of flour, one cup of butter, four eggs, two teaspoonsful of soda, a little salt. Bake in a quick oven.

WHITE CAKE.

One pound of white sugar, three-quarters of a pound of flour, six ounces of butter, the whites of fourteen eggs, beaten to a stiff froth, a little mace and citron. This cake should be frosted.

QUEEN CAKE.

Beat one pound of butter to a cream, with some rose-water, one quart of flour, and one pound of sifted sugar. Beat all well together; add a few currants, washed and dried. Bake in a moderate oven, and dredge with white sugar.

SCOTCH QUEEN CAKE.

Melt a pound of butter. Then set it away to cool. Sift two quarts of oat-meal into a pan, and mix with it a pound of powdered sugar, and a tablespoonful of powdered cinnamon and mace. Make a hole in the middle, put in the melted butter, and mix with a knife till you have formed of the whole a lump of dough. If it is too stiff, moisten it with a little rose-water. Knead it well, and roll it out into a large oval sheet, an inch thick. Cut it down the middle, and then across, so as to divide it into four cakes. Prick them with a fork, and crimp or scollop the edges neatly. Lay them in shallow pans; set them in a quick oven, and bake them of a light brown. This cake will keep a week or two. You may mix in with the dough a half-pound of currants, picked, washed, and dried.

SCOTCH CAKE.

Rub three-quarters of a pound of butter into a pound of sifted flour; mix in a pound of powdered sugar, and a large tablespoonful of powdered cinnamon. Mix it into a dough, with three well-beaten eggs. Roll it out into a sheet; cut it in round cakes, and bake them in a quick oven; they will require but a few minutes to bake.

CUP CAKE, NO. I.

Five eggs; two large teacupsful each of molasses, fine rolled brown sugar, butter, and rich milk; five cups of sifted flour; half a cup of powdered allspice and cloves, and half a cup of ginger; cut up the butter in the milk, and warm them slightly; warm also the molasses, and stir it into the milk and butter; then stir in, gradually, the sugar, and set it away to cool. Beat the eggs very light, and stir them into the mixture alternately with the flour; add the ginger and other spice, and stir the whole very hard. Butter small tins, nearly fill them with the mixture, and bake the cake in a moderate oven.

CUP CAKE, NO. II.

Take two cups of sugar, one of butter, four eggs; half a teacup of milk, half a teaspoonful of soda, four cups of flour; beat up the sugar and butter together, next add the eggs, then the flour. Beat all well together; bake quickly.

CUP CAKE, NO. III.

Nine cups of flour, four of sugar, two of butter, half a cup of milk, two teaspoonsful of soda, eight eggs, and nutmeg to the taste.

CREAM CUP CAKES.

Four cups of flour, two of sugar, three of cream, and four eggs. Beat together well, and bake in square tin pans; when cold, cut in squares, and bake in a quick oven.

CREAM CAKES.

Mix the yolks of two eggs, well beaten, with a pint of cream, two ounces of sifted sugar, a little nutmeg, cinnamon, and mace. Rub the pan with a bit of butter, and fry the pancakes.

SPONGE GINGERBREAD.

Take a piece of butter the size of a hen's egg; melt and mix it with a pint of good molasses, a quart of flour, and a spoonful of sugar; the same of ginger. Dissolve a spoonful of soda in a tumbler of milk; strain and mix it with the other ingredients, adding sufficient flour to roll out easily. Bake on flat tins in a quick oven, after rolling it out about an inch thick.

SUGAR GINGERBREAD.

Mix, with six ounces of butter, a pound of sugar; stir into this mixture four well-beaten eggs, with three teaspoonsful of ginger; add, gradually, a pound and a half of flour; dissolve a teaspoonful of soda in a wine-glass of milk; stir it in, and bake immediately.

HARD MOLASSES GINGERBREAD.

Mix a teacup of melted butter with a pint of molasses, a quart of flour, and a spoonful of ginger; dissolve a spoonful of soda in a tumbler of water; stir it in, adding enough flour to roll it out. Bake in an oven moderately warm.

SOFT MOLASSES GINGERBREAD.

Mix, with a pint of molasses, a teacup of melted butter, a pint of flour, two well-beaten eggs, and a spoonful of ginger; the peel of a fresh lemon cut into small chips is an improvement; dissolve in a tumbler of milk, and stir in two teaspoonsful of soda; add flour to make it the consistency of unbaked pound-cake. Bake about half an hour in deep pans.

GINGERBREAD CAKE.

Take three pounds of flour, one pound of sugar, one pound of butter rubbed in very fine, two ounces of ground ginger, a large nutmeg grated; then take a pound of treacle, and a quarter of a pint of cream; make them warm together; adding a spoonful of saleratus will improve them: make up the bread stiff; roll it out, and make it up into thin cakes; cut them out with a teacup or small glass, or roll them round like nuts, and bake them on tin plates in a slack oven.

SOFT GINGERBREAD.

Four teacups of flour, two cups of molasses, half a cup of butter, two cups of buttermilk, a cup of thick cream, three eggs, one tablespoonful of ground ginger, and the same of saleratus. Mix them all together, with the exception of the buttermilk, in which the saleratus must be dissolved, and then add to the rest. It must not stand long before sent to bake.

GINGER COOKIES.

Take one cup of sugar, one of molasses, one of butter, one egg, one spoonful of soda, one of ginger, and one of vinegar; add seven cups of flour.

GINGER SNAPS, NO. I.

Take one pint of molasses, one teacup of butter, one spoonful of ginger, and one teaspoonful of soda. Boil all the ingredients together. When nearly cold, add enough flour to make a soft dough.

GINGER SNAPS, NO. II.

Mix four ounces of lard, and four of butter, with four ounces of brown sugar, a pint of molasses, two spoonsful of ginger, and a quart of flour; add two teaspoonsful of soda, dissolved in a cup of buttermilk, and sufficient flour to make a soft dough; cut into small cakes, and bake in a slow oven.

RAIL-ROAD CAKE.

Six eggs, two cups of flour, two cups of sugar, one large tablespoonful of butter, four spoonsful of sweet milk, two teaspoonsful of cream of tartar, one teaspoonful of soda. Mix the cream of tartar with the flour; add the soda with the milk. Bake in a quick oven.

WINE CAKE.

Put six ounces of sugar in a pint of wine; make it boiling hot; when it has cooled to blood-heat, pour it on six well-beaten eggs, and stir in a quarter of a pound of flour; beat well, and bake immediately.

SOFT CAKE FOR TEA.

Beat ten eggs light, and one and a half pounds of sugar, a half pound of butter, two pounds of flour, a glass of rose-water, and half a nutmeg.

TEA CAKE.

Three eggs, three cups of sugar, two of butter, one of sour milk, and one and a half teaspoonsful of soda; add enough flour to make a very soft dough; roll out pretty thin, and bake in a moderate oven.

TEA CAKE—ANOTHER.

Beat to a cream, one cup of butter, with two of sugar; stir in two well-beaten eggs; add enough flour to make a soft dough; a grated nutmeg; one teaspoonful of soda dissolved in a cup of sour milk; roll out, and bake in a moderate oven.

NAPLES BISCUIT.

One pound and a half each of flour and sugar; nine eggs, half a pint of rose-water. Beat the eggs well; put the rose-water in by degrees; then mix the flour and sugar together.

SUGAR BISCUIT.

Three pounds of flour sifted, one pound of butter, a pound and a half of powdered sugar, half a pint of milk, two tablespoonsful of brandy, a small teaspoonful of pearlash dissolved in water, four tablespoonsful of caraway seeds; put the butter into the flour, add the sugar and caraway seeds, pour in the brandy, and then the milk; lastly, put in the pearlash; stir all well with a knife, and mix it thoroughly till it becomes a lump of dough; flour your paste board, and lay the dough on it; knead it very well; divide it into eight or ten pieces, and knead each piece separately; then put them all together, and knead them very well in one lump; cut the dough in half, and roll it out in sheets about half an inch thick; beat the sheets of dough very hard on both sides with the rolling-pin; cut them out into round cakes with the edge of a tumbler; butter iron pans and lay the cakes in them: bake them of a very pale brown. If done too much, they will lose their taste. These cakes, kept in a stone jar, closely covered from the air, will continue perfectly good for several months.

RUSK.

Take at night one teacup of milk, half a cup of butter, one teacup of fresh yeast, and two eggs; beat all well together; then add enough flour to make a very soft dough. In the morning, add sugar and cinnamon to the taste, and a little more flour, to have it about the consistence of loaf bread; knead it well; let it rise again; then bake with gradual heat.

RICH SMALL CAKES.

Three eggs, three tablespoonsful of butter, three of sugar, three cups of flour, one teaspoonful of essence of lemon, and half a nutmeg; work all together; roll thin; cut into small cakes, and bake.

BUNNS.

One pound and a half of flour, (a quarter of a pound left to sift in last,) half a pound of butter cut up fine together; then add four eggs; beat up to a high froth four teacups of milk, half a wine-glass of brandy, wine, and rose-water, each, and one wine-glass of yeast. Stir it all together with a knife, and add half a pound of sugar. Then sift in the quarter of a pound of flour, and when the lumps are all beaten fine, set them to rise in the pans they are to be baked in. This quantity will make four square pans full.

LOAF CAKE.

Two quarts of flour, half a pound of sugar, a quarter of a pound of butter, three eggs, one gill of milk, one half teacupful of good yeast, and cloves and nutmeg to the taste.

FRIED CAKES

One quart of milk, half a pound of butter, six eggs, and two pounds of sugar; one pound of raisins, one teaspoonful of soda, and as much flour as will make a stiff batter. Beat well, and fry in lard; take up the batter by spoonsful, and drop it in the hot lard. Each spoonful makes a cake.

DOUGHNUTS.

To one pound of flour, put one quarter of a pound of butter, one quarter of a pound of sugar, and two spoonsful of yeast; mix them all together in warm milk or water, to the thickness of bread; let it rise, and make them in what form you please; boil your lard, and put them in.

CRULLERS.

Ten eggs, one pound and a half of sugar, three-fourths of a pound of butter, one teacup of milk, one teaspoonful of saleratus, spice to your taste, and flour enough to make soft dough; let your lard be boiling, then make them into what shape you please, and put them in.

ANOTHER.

Two eggs, two teacups of sugar, two of buttermilk, with a teaspoonful of soda dissolved in it; a piece of butter the size of an egg; add enough flour to make a soft dough, and a grated nutmeg. Fry in hot lard, after rolling and cutting in any shape you prefer.

RICE PUFFS.

Four eggs, two cups of rice, cooked soft, one spoonful of butter, one cup of sour milk, one teaspoonful of soda, and three spoonsful of flour. Beat the eggs separately and very light, leaving the whites to be added just before the batter is fried. Have boiling lard to fry in; drop in one spoonful for each puff, and fry them a light brown. Lay them on a napkin to drip well before sending to table, but keep them well covered, that they may remain hot.

SODA CAKES.

Four cups of flour; three of sugar; one of butter; one of milk; five eggs; one teaspoonful of cream of tartar; half a teaspoonful of soda; nutmeg and fruit to the taste. Add the milk just before baking.

WAFER CAKES.

Mix together half a pound of powdered sugar, and a quarter of a pound of butter; and add to them six eggs well beaten. Then beat the whole very light; stirring into it as much sifted flour as will make a stiff batter; a powdered nutmeg, a teaspoonful of cinnamon; and eight drops of oil of lemon, or a tablespoonful of rose-water. The batter must be very smooth when it is done, and without a single lump. Heat your wafer-iron on both sides by turning it in the fire; but do not allow it to get too hot. Grease the inside with butter tied in a rag, (this must be repeated previous to the baking of every cake) and put in the batter, allowing to each wafer two large spoonsful.

BONIFIADAS OR STICKYS.

Make a nice soft dough as for biscuit, roll it out quite thin, and have ready prepared an equal quantity of sugar and butter melted, with enough nutmeg or cinnamon to flavor highly. Spread this mixture thick enough to cover the dough well, then commence at one side and roll it over light, until there are three thicknesses of the dough; cut it through the whole length, then cut again into cakes about two inches long; lay them in an earthen baking-dish very closely, and bake in a pretty quick oven.

This is a cheap, but a very nice cake.

LOVE CAKES.

Mix with twelve eggs, a glass of rose-water; four ounces of bitter almonds finely pounded; sugar sufficient to make a batter stiff enough to bake in paper boxes.

ELIZABETH CAKE.

A cup of butter, three of sugar, one of new milk; four eggs, a teaspoonful of soda; half a teaspoonful of cream of tartar, four cups of flour.

INDIAN POUND CAKE.

Eight eggs; the weight of eight eggs of powdered sugar; the weight of six eggs of sifted Indian-meal; half a pound of butter; one grated nutmeg, or a teaspoonful of cinnamon; stir the butter and sugar to a cream; beat the eggs very light; stir the meal and eggs alternately, into the butter and sugar; grate in the nutmeg, and stir all well. Butter a tin pan, put in the mixture, and bake it in a moderate oven.

CROQUETTES.

Take a pound of powdered sugar, a pound of butter, half a pound of wheat flour, and half a pound of Indian-meal; mix all together, and add the juice and grated peel of a large lemon, with spice to your taste. Make it into a lump of paste; then put it into a mortar, and beat it hard on all sides; roll it out thin and cut it into cakes with the edge of a tumbler, or with a tin cutter; flour a shallow tin pan; lay the cakes into it, but not close together; bake them about ten minutes; grate sugar over them when done.

MARGUERITES.

Beat together till very light, a pound of butter, and a pound of powdered sugar; sift a pound of flour into a pan; take the yolks only, of twelve eggs, and beat them till very thick and smooth. Pour them into the flour, and add the beaten butter and sugar; stir in a grated nutmeg, and a wine-glass of rose-water; mix the whole together, till it becomes a lump of dough; flour your paste board, and lay the dough upon it; sprinkle it with flour; roll it out about half an inch thick, and cut it into round cakes with the edge of a cup; flour a shallow pan, put in the cakes (so as not to touch), and bake them about five minutes in a quick oven. If the oven is too cool, they will run. When the cakes are cool, lay on each a large lump of currant-jelly: take the whites of the eggs, and beat them till they stand alone, then add to them by degrees, sufficient powdered sugar to make the consistence of icing, and ten drops of strong essence of lemon. Heap on each cake, with a spoon, a pile of the icing over the currant-jelly; set them in a cool oven till the icing becomes firm and of a pale brownish tint. These cakes are very fine.

JUMBLES.

Three eggs, half a pound of flour sifted, half a pound of butter, half a pound of powdered loaf-sugar, a tablespoonful of rose-water, a nutmeg grated, a tea-spoonful of mace and cinnamon; stir the butter and sugar to a cream, beat the eggs very light, and throw them all at once into the pan of flour; then put in the butter and sugar, and add the spice and rose-water. If you have no rose-water, six or seven drops of strong essence of lemon will answer, or more if the essence be weak: stir the whole very hard, and flour your hands well: take up with your knife a portion of the dough, and lay it on the board; roll it lightly with your hands into long thin rolls, which must be cut into equal lengths, curled up into rings, and laid gently into an iron or tin pan, buttered, not too close to each other, as they spread in baking. Bake them in a quick oven about five minutes, and grate loaf-sugar over them when cool.

PLAIN JUMBLES.

Rub eight ounçes of butter, and twelve of sugar to a cream; mix it with a pound of flour, adding a little rose-water.

MACAROONS.

Blanch and pound, with a little rose-water, a pound of sweet almonds; beat to a froth the whites of seven eggs, add to them a pound of sugar. Drop them on white paper with a spoon, and bake on tin plates, in a slow oven. Let them get cold before taking off the paper.

KISSES.

One pound of the best loaf-sugar, powdered and sifted. The whites of four eggs. Twelve drops of essence of lemon. A teacup of currant-jelly. Beat the whites of four eggs till they stand alone. Then beat in, gradually, the sugar, a teaspoonful at a time. Add the essence of lemon, and beat the whole very hard.

Lay a wet sheet of paper on the bottom of a square tin pan. Drop on it, at equal distances, a little of the beaten egg and sugar, and then add on each, a small teaspoonful of stiff currant-jelly. Then with a large spoon, pile some of the beaten egg and sugar on each lump of jelly, so as to cover it entirely. Drop on the mixture as evenly as possible, so as to make the kisses of a round smooth shape.

Set them in a cool oven, and as soon as they are colored, they are done. Then take them out and place them two bottoms together. Lay them lightly on a sieve, and dry them in a cool oven, till the two bottoms stick fast together, so as to form one ball or oval.

ICEING FOR CAKE.

Beat the whites of four eggs; then add gradually about a pound and a quarter of loaf-sugar well pulverized, beating it about half an hour; thin it with a little rose-water, if too thick to run. The cake should be almost cold before iceing. Set it in a cool oven to dry.

PUDDINGS, PIES, &c.

RULES TO BE OBSERVED IN MAKING PUDDING.

In boiled puddings take great care that the bag or cloth be very clean, and not soapy. It should be dipped in boiling water, squeezed dry, and floured before using. If a bread pudding, it should be tied loose; if a batter pudding, tie it close. The water should boil quick when the pudding is put in, and it should be moved about for a minute or two, lest the ingredients should not mix. Batter puddings should be strained through a coarse sieve when all is mixed. Where a pudding is baked, the pans and basins should be always buttered.

Very good puddings may be made without eggs, but they must have as little milk as will mix, and must boil three or four hours. A spoonful or two of yeast will answer instead of eggs.

RICE PUDDING, NO. I.

One quart of milk, four ounces of rice, one teaspoonful of cinnamon, four teaspoonsful of rose-water, eight eggs, and half a nutmeg. Boil the rice and cinnamon with the milk, and stir often to keep it from burning; after it is boiled and cooled, add the nutmeg and other spices, &c. Having beaten the eggs well, cover a deep dish with puff paste, and pour the composition in. Bake one hour and a half. Serve with butter and sugar sauce.

RICE PUDDING, NO. II.

Six pounds of rice, one quart of milk, one pound of butter, half a pound of raisins, sugar and spices to the taste. Boil the rice in the milk over a slow fire, until tender; then stir in the butter, and let it cool; beat the eggs well, and after the rice cools, put all together, and bake as No. 1.

RICE PUDDING, NO. III.

Eight spoonsful of rice, eight eggs, two quarts of milk, six ounces of butter, one pound of raisins, one nutmeg, and sugar and cinnamon to the taste. Boil the rice until soft; then add the milk and let it cool; beat the sugar with the eggs, and mix all well together.

RICE PUDDING, NO. IV.

Two quarts of milk, half a pound of rice, half a pound of raisins, one teaspoonful of cinnamon; butter and sugar to the taste.

CAROLINA RICE PUDDING.

Take half a pound of rice; wash it clean; put it into a saucepan, with a quart of milk; keep stirring it till it is very thick; take great care it does not burn; then turn it into a pan, and grate some nutmeg into it; add two teaspoonsful of beaten cinnamon and a little lemon-peel made fine. Mix all together with the yolk of three eggs, and sweeten to your taste. Then tie it up close in a cloth; put it into boiling water, and be sure to keep it boiling all the time. An hour and a quarter will be sufficient. Melt butter and pour over it, and throw some fine sugar all over it. A little wine in the sauce will be a great addition to it.

HOMINY PUDDING.

An excellent pudding may be made as follows: — Take half a pint of fine hominy, soak it one night; in the morning boil it two hours, and then proceed the same as in making a rice pudding; the addition of an egg or two improves it.

GREEN CORN PUDDING, NO. I.

Take four ears of green corn; boil them until half done; cut off the corn as fine as convenient; mix it with two spoonsful of wheat flour, one pint of sweet milk, salt and pepper to season. Bake it well.

GREEN CORN PUDDING, NO. II.

Grate sweet green corn, and to three cups of it add two quarts of milk, eight eggs, a grated nutmeg, two teaspoonsful of salt, and six ounces of drawn butter. Bake one hour.

GREEN CORN PUDDING, NO. III.

Cut the corn from the cob, and pound it fine. To four dozen ears add a pint of milk, and half a pound of sugar. Mix, and bake about two hours, till the crust is a dark brown. Eat with butter, to which some add a little pepper.

BAKED INDIAN PUDDING, NO. I.

One quart of milk, five large tablespoonsful of Indian-meal, four eggs, nutmeg and sugar to the taste. Boil the milk; scald the meal in it; then let it cool before you add the eggs. Bake three-quarters of an hour, in a moderate oven.

BAKED INDIAN PUDDING, NO. II.

Boil one quart of milk; mix with it, perfectly smooth, two gills and a half of Indian-meal; then add seven eggs, well-beaten, a gill of molasses, a spoonful of butter. Bake two hours, in a moderate oven.

BAKED INDIAN PUDDING, NO. III.

Take one quart of corn meal, two quarts of warm milk, about blood-heat, two teaspoonsful of salt, one teacup of molasses, or four tablespoonsful of sugar, one tablespoonful of chopped suet, and half a grated nutmeg. Bake this mixture in a pan two hours.

BAKED INDIAN PUDDING, NO. IV.

Take fourteen tablespoonsful of Indian-meal, two quarts of boiling milk, two teaspoonsful of salt, and half a tablespoonful of chopped suet. A richer pudding is made by substituting for the fourteen tablespoonsful of Indian-meal, seven eggs and only seven tablespoonsful of meal.

The sauce may consist of one pint of water, four tablespoonsful of sugar, butter the size of half an egg, one tablespoonful of vinegar, one tablespoonful of flour, and a quarter of a nutmeg. It should be boiled three or four minutes.

RICH INDIAN PUDDING—BAKED.

Boil a quart of milk, add a pint of fine Indian-meal. Stir it well. Mix three tablespoonsful of wheat flour with a pint of milk, so as to have it free from lumps. Mix this with the meal, and stir the whole well together. When the whole is moderately warm, stir in three eggs well beat, with three spoonsful of sugar. Add two teaspoonsful of salt, two of ground cinnamon, or grated nutmegs, and two tablespoonsful of melted butter. When the pudding has baked five or six minutes, stir in half a pound of raisins, seeded; and add half a pint of milk for them, as they will otherwise render it too dry. Bake three or four hours.

BOILED INDIAN PUDDING, NO. I.

Make a stiff batter, by stirring Indian-meal into a quart of boiling milk or water. Then stir in two tablespoonsful of flour, three of sugar, half a spoonful of ginger, or two teaspoonsful of cinnamon, and two teaspoonsful of salt, two tablespoonsful of fine chopped suet. Such puddings require a long boiling, say seven or eight hours. They require good sauce for eating.

BOILED INDIAN PUDDING, NO. II.

One teacup of molasses, a piece of suet the size of two eggs, chopped fine, eight spoonsful of meal. Scald the meal with boiling water or milk; mix it quite thin; when it is nearly cold, add four eggs, well beaten. It requires three hours' boiling, in a strong cloth.

LEMON PUDDING, NO. I.

Half a pound of sugar, half a pound of butter, one lemon, five eggs, a wineglass of rose-water, the same of orange-flower water. Beat the rose-water and butter to a froth; prepare the sugar and eggs as for a pound-cake; grate the yellow part of the lemon-rind in. Have a nice puff paste ready in your dish; and after mixing your pudding well together, put it into the paste. Bake in a moderate oven. Orange pudding is made in the same way, using a pounded orange instead of a lemon.

LEMON PUDDING, NO. II.

Three lemons, eight eggs, half a pound of sugar, one wine-glass of rose or orange water, four ounces of Naples' biscuit, one quart of milk or cream, one pound of fresh butter. Cut the rinds of the lemons; boil them tender in water; then pound them in a mortar. Boil up the biscuit in the milk, beat the eggs and sugar together, and mix all well together. Stir it over the fire till quite thick, squeeze in the juice of a large lemon, put puff paste over the dish, then pour in the pudding. Cut candied sweetmeats and strew over the top.

YORKSHIRE PUDDING.

Beat up four eggs, and mix with them, by degrees, four spoonsful of flour; beat it to a smooth paste, and add a pint of new milk and a little salt. Put it into a shallow square tin, under roast meat. It should not be put down until the meat is warmed through, and begins to drip. The tin should be very warm when the pudding is put in, to keep the floury part from settling.

ORANGE PUDDING.

Grate the yellow part of a smooth, deep-colored orange, and of a lime, into a saucer, and squeeze in their juice, taking out the seeds. Stir four ounces of butter, and four of powdered sugar, to a cream. Beat three eggs as light as possible, and stir them gradually into the pan of butter and sugar; add gradually a spoonful of brandy and wine, and a teaspoonful of rose-water; then the orange and lime all together. Have prepared a sheet of puff paste, made of five ounces of flour and four ounces of fresh butter; spread the sheet in a pudding-pan, trim and notch the edges, and then turn in the mixture. Bake it about thirty minutes, in a moderate oven. Grate loaf-sugar over it.

MINUTE PUDDING.

Six gills of wheat or rye flour, two gills of milk, half a nutmeg, and a teaspoonful of salt. When the milk boils, turn in the other ingredients: let the whole boil for one minute, stirring it constantly; then move it from the fire, and on its becoming luke-warm, add three beaten eggs. Set it on the fire again, stir constantly till it thickens, and remove it as soon as it boils.

TURKEY PUDDING.

Mince thirty small onions, and mix them with an equal quantity of bread crumbs that have been soaked in milk. Chop an equal quantity of the flesh of cold turkey; mix all together, and pound it very well in a mortar. Pass it through a colander, and then return it to the mortar and beat it again, adding gradually the yolks of six hard eggs, and a pint of cream, or half a pound of butter; season it to your taste with salt, mace and nutmeg. Have ready some skins, nicely cleaned as for sausages; fill the skins with the mixture, and tie up the ends. Then simmer your puddings, but do not let them boil. Take them out, drain them, and put them away to get cold. When you wish to cook them for immediate use, prick them with a fork, wrap them in buttered paper, and broil them on a gridiron.

MUFFIN OR CABINET PUDDING.

Cut three or four muffins in two; pour over them boiling milk sufficient to cover them; let them remain in it until they are tender. Make a rich custard with eight eggs (leaving out four whites), a pint of cream, a quarter of a pound of loaf-sugar, an ounce of almonds blanched and cut, lemon-peel and nutmeg grated, and a glass of brandy. Butter a tin mold, for boiling — or, for baking, a dish. Put in a layer of dried cherries, green gages, apricots, or French plums; cover with custard, add more fruit, then custard, until the mold or dish is full. Boil an hour and a half, and serve with wine sauce. The mold should not float in the water, but stand in a stew-pan, with only water enough to reach half-way up it. Baking will not take so long. Lay a puff paste round the edges of the dish.

SWISS PUDDING.

Put layers of crumbs of bread and sliced apples, with sugar between, until the dish is full; let crumbs be the uppermost layer; then pour milk over it, and bake.

OXFORD PUDDING.

Take a quarter of a pound of grated biscuit, the same quantity of currants, the same of suet finely chopped, a spoonful of sugar, and a little nutmeg; mix them all together. Add the yolks of three eggs, and make up the pudding into balls. Fry them a light color, in fresh butter; and serve with white wine sauce.

FRENCH AND ITALIAN PUDDING.

These puddings are composed of sliced rolls, eggs, and cream. Five or six eggs to a pint of cream, and as much roll as will thicken it; sweeten with loaf-sugar. A pound of suet chopped fine may be added or not. Line the dish with puff-paste; lay at the bottom six or eight apples cut up, a pound of raisins stoned, a few dates sliced, some candied orange-peel, sugar, and spice. Pour the pudding over this, grate nutmeg on the top, and bake to a delicate brown.

A CHEESE PUDDING.

Half a pound of cheese grated, two ounces of butter, four eggs, a little cayenne, and nutmeg. Butter a dish, and bake twenty minutes.

A VERY RICH PUDDING OF PRIME RIPE FRUIT.

This is made sometimes by pressing the fruit through a sieve, if apricots, green gages, or peaches. Sweet, juicy apples, or rich mellow pears may be grated; or the fruit may be scalded a few minutes in white wine, then the skins and stones removed and beaten in a mortar. When cold mix with rich custard, cream, eggs, and bread-crumbs or Naples biscuit, with loaf-sugar to the taste, and a glass of brandy or Sherry wine. Bake in a dish edged with puff-paste. For these puddings the tinctures are preferable to the spices.

SWEET POTATO PUDDING.

Boil one pound of sweet potatoes very tender, rub them while hot through a colander; add six eggs well beaten, three quarters of a pound of powdered sugar, three quarters of a pound of butter, and some nutmeg and lemon-peel, with a glass of brandy; put a paste in the dish, and when the pudding is done sprinkle the top.

POTATO PUDDING, NO. I.

Twelve ounces of baked potatoes skinned and mashed, one ounce of suet, one ounce of cheese grated fine, one gill of sweet milk. Mix the potatoes, suet, and cheese all together, and if too thick, add a little water. Bake in an earthen pan.

POTATO PUDDING, NO. II.

One pound of butter, one pound of sugar, beat to a cream; one pound of potatoes, boiled and passed through the colander, eight eggs, one glass of brandy, one of wine, half a glass of rose-water, and one teaspoonful of spice.

ALMOND PUDDING.

One pound of blanched almonds, six eggs, eight ounces of sugar, one pint of cream, a half-glass of rose-water. Bake in a moderate oven.

GINGER PUDDING.

Six cups of flour, two cups of sugar, one cup of molasses, one cup of butter, two cups of butter-milk, with a teaspoonful of soda for each cup of milk, four eggs, and ginger to the taste.

CITRON PUDDING.

One pound of sugar, three quarters of a pound of butter, creamed, the beaten yolks of ten eggs, one spoonful of flour, two teaspoonsful of vinegar, and citron to the taste.

MOLASSES PUDDING.

One cup of butter, one cup of molasses, one cup of sugar, one cup of milk, one teaspoonful of soda, one tablespoonful of ginger. Bake in a moderate oven.

BATTER PUDDING.

Take a quart of milk, and stir into it gradually eight tablespoonsful of flour, carefully pressing out all the lumps with a spoon. Beat eight eggs very light, and add them by degrees to the milk and flour.

BOILED PUDDING.

Five eggs, half a pint of milk, half a tea-cup of butter or lard, same of sugar; put flour in until it is a stiff batter; rub into the batter (through a sieve,) either green or dry fruit; put into a bag and boil two hours — the water must be kept boiling hot. Sauce of butter and sugar.

COCOANUT PUDDING, NO. I.

After peeling the cocoanut, grate it, and to a pound of cocoanut add half a pound of butter, six tablespoonsful of white sugar, and the whites of a dozen eggs, well beaten. Flavor with lemon and nutmeg. Bake on a rich pastry-crust, in a slow oven.

COCOANUT PUDDING, NO. II.

Weigh three quarters of a pound of cocoanut, and grate it in a dish; cut up half a pound of butter in half a pound of white sugar, and stir them together to a cream; add to them a glass of wine and rose-water mixed; beat the whites of twelve eggs until they stand alone on the rods, and stir the grated cocoanut and the whites of the eggs alternately into the butter and sugar. Bake it in puff-paste.

TAPIOCA PUDDING.

One quart of milk, five eggs, one coffee-cup of tapioca, one half-cup of butter. Beat up the eggs with sugar, to the taste, and add a few drops of essence of lemon. Bake half an hour in a moderate oven.

PLAIN BAKED PUDDING.

Two eggs well beaten; a cup of powdered white sugar; a teaspoonful of soda dissolved in a cup of sweet milk; two teaspoonsful of cream of tartar mixed through three cups of flour; and a table-spoonful of lard or butter. Bake quickly, and serve with sugar, butter, and wine sauce.

TRANSPARENT PUDDING.

Eight eggs, eight ounces of butter, eight ounces of sugar. Beat up the eggs, put them in a stew-pan with the sugar and butter, season with nutmeg. Set it on a stove or fire of coals, stirring it constantly, until it thickens, then pour it in a basin to cool. Line your dish with a rich paste, pour your pudding in, and bake in a moderate oven.

CHESHIRE PUDDING.

One pound of raspberry jam, four ounces of butter, one tablespoonful of soda, one cup of cream or butter-milk, one half-pound of flour.

Rub half of the butter into the flour, warm the milk, rub the soda fine and pour it into the milk, and while it is effervescing pour it into the butter.

APPLE PUDDING.

Take twelve large pippins, pare them and take out the cores, put them into a saucepan with four or five spoonsful of water, boil them till they are soft and thick, then beat them well; stir in a pound of loaf-sugar, the juice of three lemons cut thin and beat fine in a mortar, the yolks of eight eggs beaten; mix all well together; bake it in a slack oven; when it is near done throw over a little fine sugar: you may bake it in a puff-paste as you do other puddings.

VIRGINIA CHICKEN PUDDING.

Beat ten eggs very light, add to them a quart of rich milk; four ounces of drawn butter; pepper and salt to the taste; stir in sufficient flour to make a thin batter; —Take four young chickens (clean them nicely and cut off the legs, wings, &c.,) put them in a sauce-pan, with salt and water; and a bundle of thyme and parsley. Boil them until nearly done, then take out the chickens and put them in the batter, in a deep dish and bake it. Serve with white gravy sauce.

PUMPKIN PUDDING.

Half a pound of butter, half a pound of sugar, beat to a cream; one pound of pumpkin stewed and passed through the colander; four eggs, one wine-glass of brandy, wine, and rose-water, and one teaspoonful of spice.

CARROT PUDDING.

Grate half a pound of carrots, one pound of bread, the whites of eight eggs, half a pound of butter, half a pint of cream or milk, half a pint of wine and rose-water, and spice and sweeten to taste. Lay a puff paste over the dish. Bake one hour, and sift sugar over it.

BATH PUDDING.

Take one pint of new milk, six eggs beat well in the milk, four tablespoonsful of fine flour, three table-spoonsful of yeast, three spoonsful of rose-water, and three spoonsful of Malaga wine; grate into it a small nutmeg; sweeten with fine sugar to your taste; mix them all well together, and let them stand one hour before they are to be baked: bake them in eight small patty-pans, and one large one for the middle of the dish: butter the patty-pans; put them in a hot oven, and in fifteen minutes they will be done.

QUAKING PUDDING.

Take a pint of good cream, six eggs, and half the whites; beat them well, and mix with the cream; grate in a small nutmeg; add a little rose-water if it be desired; grate in the crust of a small loaf of bread, or add a spoonful or two of flour first mixed with a little of the cream, or a spoonful of the flour of rice, which you please; butter a cloth well and flour it; then put in your mixtures; tie it not too close, and boil it half an hour: be sure the water boils before you put it in.

BREAD PUDDING.

Take the crumbs of a small loaf of bread, and as much flour; the yolks of four eggs and two whites, a teaspoonful of ginger; half a pound of raisins, seeded; half a pound of currants, clean washed and picked, and a little salt; mix first the bread and flour, ginger, salt, and sugar to your taste; then the eggs, and as much milk as will make it like a good batter; butter the dish; pour it in, and bake it.

RICH BREAD AND BUTTER PUDDING.

Cut a pound loaf of good bread into thin slices; spread them with butter as for eating; lay them in a pudding dish; sprinkle between each layer of bread seeded raisins, and citron cut fine; beat eight eggs with four tablespoonsful of rolled sugar; mix them with three pints of milk, and half a grated nutmeg. Turn the whole on the bread in the pan, and let it remain till the bread has taken up full half the milk; then bake about three quarters of an hour.

PLUM PUDDING.

Beat eight eggs very light; add one pint of milk, one quart of flour, and three-quarters of a pound of butter; cut and stone half a pound of raisins, and mix them in the batter with half a nutmeg grated; wet the cloth, and tie it tight; put the pudding in when the water boils, and shake it a minute or two to keep the raisins from settling. Boil two hours.

NORFOLK PUDDING.

Make a thick batter, as you would for pancakes; take half a pint of milk, two eggs, a little salt, and make it into a batter with flour; have ready a clean saucepan of water boiling, into which drop the batter. Be sure the water boils fast, and two or three minutes will boil them; then throw them into a sieve or colander to drain the water away; then turn them into a dish, and stir a lump of fresh butter into them; eat them hot, and they are very good.

CUSTARD PUDDING.

One quart of milk, six eggs, six spoonsful of flour. Boil the milk, and while boiling stir in the flour; set it to cool half an hour before it is used; Beat up the eggs nicely, and then stir in the other ingredients. Bake in a moderate oven about 25 minutes.

BAKED CUSTARD.

Two quarts of milk, twelve eggs, twelve ounces of sugar, one nutmeg. Bake in pans.

PLAIN CUSTARDS.

A quart of rich milk, eight eggs, a quarter of a pound of powdered sugar, a handful of peach leaves, or half an ounce of peach kernels broken fine, and a nutmeg. Boil the peach leaves or kernels in the milk, and set it away to cool. When cold, strain out the leaves or kernels, and stir in the sugar. Beat the eggs very light, and stir them gradually into the milk when it is quite cold. Bake it in cups, or in a large white dish. When cool, grate nutmeg over the top.

CUP CUSTARD.

To every teacup of milk add one egg; one tablespoonful of sugar; flavor with lemon, and eat cold. Eight eggs will fill a dozen glasses.

RASPBERRY DUMPLINGS.

Make a puff paste, and roll it out; spread the raspberry jam, and make it into dumplings; boil them an hour; pour melted butter into a dish, and strew grated sugar over them.

BAKED APPLE DUMPLINGS.

Make a short crust, and divide into small pieces, made thin and round; have ready pared and cored as many apples as you wish to make into dumplings, allowing one apple to each. After putting in the apple, fill up the cavity from whence the core was taken, with sugar, butter, and a little cinnamon; close up the crust to make it round and smooth; lay them in a deep baking-dish, which you will fill nearly full of a rich sauce, made of water, sugar, butter, and cinnamon. Bake in a moderate oven, and have enough syrup to keep the dumplings well covered, and to allow a spoonful to pour over each one when they are served at dinner.

BOILED APPLE DUMPLINGS.

Take a good puff paste; pare some large apples; cut them into quarters, and take out the cores very nicely; take a piece of crust and roll it large enough for one apple; roll the crust round each apple, and make them round like a ball, with a little flour in your hand; have a pot of water boiling; take a clean cloth, dip it in the water, and shake flour over it; tie each dumpling by itself, and put them in the water boiling all the time; and if your crust is light and good, and the apples not too large, half an hour will boil them; but if the apples are large, they will take an hour boiling. When they are boiled enough, take them up and lay them in a dish and send them to the table; have good fresh butter melted with sugar, mixed for sauce.

RISSOLES.

Make some puff paste, and cut it out with the edge of a tumbler; have ready some seasoned minced veal, or some chopped oysters, or any kind of forcemeat, and lay some of it on one-half of each piece of paste; then turn over it the other half, so as to enclose the meat; crimp the edges; put some butter into a frying-pan; lay the rissoles into it, and fry them a light brown. They should be in the shape of a half-moon.

VEAL PIE.

Cut into steaks, a loin or breast of veal; season them highly, with pepper, salt, grated nutmeg, mace, and lemon peel; lay them in the bottom of a dish, and then a few slices of sweet-breads; add some oysters, a tablespoonful of lemon-pickle, forcemeat balls, hard-boiled eggs, and a half-pint of white stock. Put puff paste on a dish, and put the pie on it; cover with puff paste, and bake one hour in a slow oven.

MUTTON PIE.

Cut the mutton into slices, without bone; season highly, and stew it with some fat, cut into slices also. It is not necessary to add any water. When tender, take it from the fire, and allow it to remain in the oven until cold; remove all the grease and fat very carefully; have some gravy made from the bones; add to it strained gravy from the mutton, and a glass of port-wine. A minced shallot and button onions are a good addition; and if the latter be pickled, their acidity will be an improvement. Put it into a dish or small patty-pans, using puff paste. These pies are better hot than cold. The underdone part of a leg of mutton may be thus dressed, but the loin and kidney are better suited for the purpose.

BEEFSTEAK PIE.

Choose steak that has long been hung; cut it into moderately sized pieces, and trim off all the skin and sinews; season them with pepper, salt, and minced shallot or onion; lay them in a dish, which should have a nice crust in it; put in enough water and butter to make a nice gravy; cover it with a thick crust, and bake it an hour with moderate heat.

LOBSTER PIE.

Having boiled the lobster, take out the meat from the shell, season it with salt, mustard, cayenne pepper, and vinegar, and beat it well in a mortar. Then stir in a quarter of a pound of butter, the yolks of two beaten eggs, and two ounces or more of grated bread crumbs. Make some puff paste, put in the mixture, and cover it with a lid of paste ornamented with leaves or flowers of the same. Bake it slowly.

SWEET POTATO CUSTARD PIE.

To one pound of potatoes, baked and sifted, add half a pound of butter, three quarters of a pound of sugar, one pint of milk, and six eggs; flavor with nutmeg, cinnamon, and a wine-glass of brandy. Line your dish with a nice pastry-crust, and bake with moderate heat.

POTATO CUSTARD PIE.

To one pound of potatoes, (mashed and strained), add three quarters of a pound of butter, twelve eggs beaten separately; one quart of sweet milk; and one pound of sugar. Flavor with nutmeg and cinnamon.

GREEN APPLE CUSTARD PIE.

Peel and core your apples, stew them quickly in enough water to prevent them from burning. When done, mash and strain them, and to a quart of fruit add four eggs well beaten, one pint of sweet milk, four ounces of melted butter, a nutmeg, a teaspoonful of lemon-juice, and a half-pound of light sugar. Let your apples cool before you add the eggs, &c. Bake in rich pastry crusts.

DRIED APPLE CUSTARD PIE.

After stewing your apples in water until perfectly done, strain them, and sweeten to your taste; then put it into pastry crusts in deep shapes or plates; also have prepared the following mixture: — For a quart of apples, four eggs, one pint of sweet milk, half a pound of sugar, one spoonful of melted butter, a nutmeg, and a teaspoonful of lemon-juice. Pour it on the tops of your custards thick enough to cover them well. Beat the mixture well before putting it on the apples. Bake in a moderate oven.

APPLE CUSTARD PIE, NO. I.

Take the weight of ten eggs in sugar, the same of stewed apples, half the weight of butter; use only half the eggs, and season with nutmeg. The same receipt is equally good for potatoes.

APPLE CUSTARD PIE, NO. II.

Four sweet apples grated, three pints of milk, two eggs, sugar to the taste, and flavor with nutmeg or lemon. Bake with two crusts.

LEMON PIE.

Take one lemon, slice it very thin, lay it in a rich paste, sprinkle over it one spoonful of flour, one tea-cup of sugar. Fill the pie nearly full of water, and cover. Bake in a slow oven nearly an hour.

RED SUGAR-BEET PIE.

Pies made of red sugar-beet are delicious, somewhat resembling rhubarb pie in flavor, though more rich and substantial. Season with vinegar, sugar, and spices to suit the taste; the root may be used without boiling if chopped fine, though I would recommend boiling first. Bake as you would an apple pie.

MINCE PIE.

Take beef tongue, weighing about three pounds, cut off the root, wash it perfectly clean, and boil it till it becomes tender; skin it, and when cold, chop it very finely. Or, if preferred, three pounds of the inside of a sirloin of beef, boiled till it becomes tender, and chopped finely as the other. Mince, as small as possible, two pounds of fresh beef suet; two pounds of currants, nicely picked, washed, rubbed, and dried at the fire; two dozen large apples, pared and chopped very fine; one pound of good brown sugar; sift half an ounce of mace, and a quarter of an ounce of cloves; grate in two nutmegs. The grated rind and juice of a large lemon may be added, with a little citron. Put all together into a large pan, and mix it well together with half a pint of good French brandy, and if not moist enough, good sweet cider may be added. Put it down close into a jar, covered closely, and it will be good four months. When you make your pies, take small round dishes, or soup-plates; lay a thin crust all over them, put in your meat, lay over the crust, and bake them nicely. If the meat is not to be used immediately, the apples had better not be put in until wanted.

PUMPKIN PIE, NO. I.

Take one quart of stewed and strained pumpkin; add one quart of new milk, half a pint of cream, and four eggs well beaten. Mix, and add a little ginger, cinnamon, and sugar, to the taste. Put a bottom crust of puff paste, and bake in deep dishes.

PUMPKIN PIE, NO. II.

To one quart of stewed and strained pumpkin, add one quart of new milk, and sweeten to the taste. For the crust, take wheat flour; wet with buttermilk to a sufficient stiffness to roll out. Bake it in deep dishes.

PUMPKIN PIE, NO. III.

Take a brown earthen pan, grease it, and sift Indian-meal over it, about the thickness of a quarter of an inch. Prepare the pumpkin in good new milk, sweeten to the taste, and add a little ground rice instead of eggs, with a little ginger. Bake as above.

APPLE PIE.

Make a good puff paste crust; lay some around the sides and bottom of the dish; pare and cut your apples, and stew them; put in a thick layer of apples; throw in half the sugar you design for your pie; make a little orange-peel fine; squeeze and throw over them a little of the orange-juice, then a few cloves, then the rest of your apples and sugar. Sweeten to your taste. Boil the peelings and cores of the apples, with a blade of mace. Strain it, and boil the syrup with a little sugar, till there is but very little left. Pour it into the pie, put on the upper crust, and bake it.

CRANBERRY PIE.

Wash and stew a quart of good sound cranberries; strain them through a coarse sieve; add half a pound of good sugar. Put a bottom crust in your patty-pans, fill them up, and bake in a moderate oven for half an hour.

RHUBARB PIE.

Cut the stalks to pieces of the size of a gooseberry, stew them a little in a sauce-pan, put them into a dish covered with a crust; squeeze over them a little lemon-juice, adding orange-peel, sugar, rose-water, and cinnamon to your taste; cover the whole with a good puff paste, and bake it.

SWEET-POTATO PIE.

Select four or five of the largest potatoes; wash them clean; slice them thin, and put in a pan with a puff paste crust, first a layer of potatoes; then season with allspice, cinnamon, sugar, and butter, and so fill up the pan, observing to put a little of the seasoning between each layer as you fill up; one good sized lemon may be cut and sliced thin, and added between each layer of the potatoes. A sufficient quantity of water must be added, so that the pie may be moist after it is baked. Cover the top with a puff paste, and bake in an oven.

TOMATO PIE.

The tomatoes are skinned and sliced, and after being mixed with sugar, are spiced and prepared in the same manner as other pies.

BLANC MANGE.

Simmer an ounce of fine isinglass in a pint and a half of new milk; add the rind of half a lemon; shred very fine a blade or two of mace and a stick of cinnamon, and sweeten with two ounces and a half of loaf-sugar. Blanch and pound with a spoonful of rose-water, half an ounce of sweet almonds, and eight or ten of bitter; put to the milk, and mix. When the isinglass is quite dissolved, strain through white flannel into half a pint of rich cream, and stir together well. When it has stood an hour, pour it off into another basin, leaving the sediments at the bottom, and when nearly cold, pour it into molds, jelly-glasses, or custard-cups. Two spoonsful of noyeau will answer the purpose of the almonds. The isinglass may be dissolved in a pint of water, and half a pint of milk.

QUINCE BLANC MANGE.

Dissolve one ounce of clarified isinglass in a pint of quince juice; add ten ounces of coarsely-powdered sugar, and stir gently over a clear fire about twenty-five minutes, or until it jellies on falling from the spoon. Skim well; then gradually pour the boiling jelly to a pint of cream, briskly stirring it until almost cold. Turn it into molds which have been dipped in cold water.

ARROW-ROOT BLANC MANGE, NO. I.

Take a teacupful of arrow-root, put it in a large bowl, and dissolve it in a little cold water. When it is melted, pour off the water, and let the arrow-root remain undisturbed. Boil it in half a pint of un-skimmed milk, made very sweet with white sugar; add a beaten nutmeg, and eight or nine blades of mace, mixed with the juice and grated peel of a lemon. When it has boiled long enough to be highly-flavored, strain it into a pint and a half of very rich milk or cream, and add a quarter of a pound of sugar. Boil the whole for ten minutes; then strain it, boiling hot, over the arrow-root. Stir it well, and frequently, till cold; then put it into molds, and let it congeal.

ARROW-ROOT BLANC MANGE, NO. II.

Put two teacupsful of arrow-root to a quart of milk. Flavor it with an ounce of sweet almonds, and fifteen or sixteen bitter almonds, blanched and pounded; or with noyeau. Moisten the arrow-root with a little cold milk, and pour in it the boiling milk, stirring all the time. Then put it in the saucepan, and boil a minute or two, still stirring.

CARRAGEEN BLANC MANGE.

This is made of a sea-weed, resembling moss. It is found in large quantities on some parts of our coast, and is sold by city druggists. Carrageen costs but little, and is considered extremely salutary for persons of delicate constitutions. Its glutinous nature, when boiled, renders it very suitable for blanc mange.

From a quart of rich unskimmed milk take half a pint. Add to it two ounces of bitter almonds, blanched and pounded, half a nutmeg, and a large stick of cinnamon broken up; also eight or nine blades of mace. Set it in a closed pan over bright coals, and boil it half an hour. In the mean time wash through two or three cold waters half a handful of carrageen (too much of it will give an unpleasant taste to the blanc mange), and add it to the pint and a half of cold milk. When it is sufficiently flavored, stir in the boiled milk, adding gradually half a pound of powdered loaf-sugar, and mix the whole well. Set it over the fire, and boil hard five minutes. Then strain it into a pitcher, wet your mold or cups with cold water, put the blanc mange into them, and leave it undisturbed until it congeals.

After washing the sea-weed, you must drain it well, and shake the water from the sprigs. You may flavor the mixture (after it is boiled and strained), with rose or peach water, stirred in last.

WHIP SYLLABUB.

Make a whip as for trifle; mix with a pint of cream, half a pint of sweet wine, the juice of a lemon, a glass of brandy, six ounces of loaf-sugar, and grated nutmeg; nearly fill the custard-cups with the mixture, and put on with a spoon some of the whip.

GOOSEBERRY OR APPLE FOOL.

Stew green gooseberries or apples, peeled and cored; add to them a little moist sugar, enough to draw the juice; to two quarts of fruit, a quarter of a pound of sugar. When quite tender, put through a coarse sieve; and if not sweet enough, add more sugar, and a quart of new milk warm from the cow (if not from the cow, warm it by the fire), a teacupful of cream, and an egg, or two yolks well beaten. Let it thicken in the milk, and be careful it does not boil. When cold, mix the fruit, and stir all well together till united.

A FRIAR'S OMELET.

Boil a dozen apples, as for sauce; stir in a quarter of a pound of butter, and the same of white sugar; when cold, add four eggs, well beaten; put it into a baking-dish, thickly strewn over with crumbs of bread, so as to stick to the bottom and sides; then put in the apple-mixture; strew crumbs of bread over the top. When baked, turn it out, and grate loaf-sugar over it.

CREAM FOR FRUIT PIES.

Simmer a pint of new milk, the rind of a lemon, and a little cinnamon; whisk the yolks of two eggs, with half a spoonful of flour, and one or two of cream; gradually add the boiling milk, set it over the fire, and whisk it till it is the consistence of thick cream. When it is removed from the fire, and rather cool, add a tablespoonful of rose or orange water.

When quite cold, take off the top of the pie and pour in the cream; return the cover, either whole, or in quarters. Rich cream may be prepared, with an equal quantity of cream and milk flavored with almond, lemon, ratafa, or brandy, and called by the name of the article with which it is principally flavored. Be careful not to let your creams boil, or they will curdle. Creams may be prepared with fresh or preserved fruits. Luscious fruits may be improved by the addition of lemon-juice.

TRIFLE.

Mix, in a large bowl, a quarter of a pound of sifted sugar, a bit of lemon-peel grated fine, and the juice of a whole lemon, half a gill of Lisbon or sweet wine, the same of brandy, and a pint and a half of good cream. Whisk the whole well, and take off the froth as it rises with a skimmer, and put it on a sieve; continue to whisk it till you have enough of the whip, and set it in a cold place to drain three or four hours. Then put in a dish eight sponge biscuit, two ounces of almonds, grated nutmeg, lemon, currant-jelly, raspberry-jam, wine and brandy to the taste. Pour over them a pint of custard, and plenty of the whip.

FLOATING ISLAND.

Take a quart of the thickest cream you can get, make it pretty sweet with fine sugar, pour in a gill of sack, grate in it the yellow rind of a lemon, and mill the cream till it is of a thick froth: then carefully pour the thin from the froth into a dish, take a French roll, or as many as you want, cut it as thin as you can, put a layer of that as light as possible on the cream; then a layer of currant-jelly, then a very thin layer of roll, and then hartshorn jelly, then French roll, and over that whip your froth which you saved of the cream, very well milled up, and lay it on top as high as you can heap it.

RICE MILK FOR A DESSERT.

Boil half a pint of rice in water till tender. Pour off the water, and add a pint of milk, with two eggs beaten and well stirred into it. Boil all together for a few minutes. Serve it up hot, and eat it with butter, sugar, and nutmeg. It may be sweetened and cooled in molds, turned out on a deep dish, and surrounded with rich milk, seasoned with wine and sugar.

APPLE COMPOTE.

Take ripe apples, pare, core and weigh them, and to each pound allow a pound of fine loaf-sugar and two lemons; parboil the apples, and set them aside to cool. Pare off very nicely, with a pen-knife, the yellow rind of the lemon, taking care not to break it, and then with scissors trim the edges to an even width all along. Put the lemon-rind to boil by itself until it becomes tender, and set it to cool.

Allow half a pint of water to each pound of sugar, and when it is melted, set it on the fire in a preserving-kettle, put in the apples, and boil till they are clear and tender all through, but do not allow them to break. Skim the syrup carefully, after you have taken out the apples, add the lemon-juice, put in the lemon-peel, and boil till quite transparent.

PRESERVES AND JELLIES.

CURRANT JELLY.

Pick the currants, put them in a stone jar, and place it to stew in a sauce-pan of boiling water till the juice is extracted. Strain through a sieve without pressing them, and boil the juice in an enamelled sauce-pan with its weight of loaf-sugar, removing the scum as it rises. When it will jelly on the back of a cold spoon, it is sufficiently done. A little of the jelly dissolved in warm water forms an agreeable beverage.

CALVES' FEET JELLY.

Boil down one set of calves' feet in four quarts of water, till it is reduced one-half, then strain through a sieve in order to remove the bones; when settled and cold, take off the grease on the surface, then boil with the following additions: — twelve eggs, three-pints of good Sherry wine, add two pounds of loaf-sugar, the juice of four lemons; stir the mixture well with a whisk, and filter through a fine flannel bag. Jellies of Champagne and other wines are made in the same way.

COFFEE JELLY.

Is made the same as the preceding, using, instead of Sherry wine, a decoction of coffee prepared as follows: — infuse half a pound of Mocha coffee, pulverised or ground, in one quart of water, strain off the decoction, and add to it a little brandy.

TEA JELLY, GREEN OR BLACK.

Treat in the same way as the foregoing, using an infusion of half an ounce of tea to one quart of water.

PRESERVED CUCUMBERS.

After greening with vine-leaves and alum, wipe the cucumbers in a dry cloth, and season the inside with a mixture of bruised mace and lemon-peel. Tie on with a pack-thread the piece that was taken out. To every pound of cucumbers, add a pound of loaf-sugar. Put them in a preserving-kettle, a half-pint of water to each pound, and the beaten white of an egg to every four pounds. Boil and skim the sugar till quite clear, adding sliced ginger and lemon to suit the taste. When cool, pour it over the cucumbers, and let them lie in it two days, keeping them covered with a plate, with a weight on it. Then boil up the syrup again adding one-half as much sugar &c., as at first, and lastly add the juice and grated peel of two lemons, for every six cucumbers. The lemon must boil in the syrup but two minutes. Then strain the syrup over the cucumbers, and put them up in small jars corded tightly.

ORANGE PRESERVES.

Choose your oranges of a fine clear skin; make a hole at the stalk end, large enough to admit the end of a spoon, with which you take out the pulp; throw them in salt and water, and let them remain three or four days; drain them from this, and put them in a pan of fresh water, and let them boil until the end of a straw may be pushed through the peel; throw them in cold water, and with the end of a spoon clear out any part of the pulp which may have adhered to them; drain off the water; put them in a tub or pan, and pour boiling syrup over them; let them remain in this three or four days; take them from the syrup, and boil it again, adding more as the peels imbibe it, so as to keep them well covered; boil the syrup once in every four or five days, and pour it hot over them; do this until it has fully penetrated them.

ORANGE JELLY.

Squeeze the juice out of twelve Havana oranges, and one lemon; strain through a fine linen cloth; then mix with the boiled syrup; add the clarified isinglass, filter through a fine flannel bag, and finish as before.

The foregoing will suffice for all fruit jellies.

ORANGE MARMALADE.

Procure some large Seville oranges with clear skins, peel them, squeeze out the pulp and juice, taking care to remove all the pips. Boil the peel (divided into quarters) till they are sufficiently tender; scrape clean all the inside from them, lay them in folds, and cut into very thin slices about an inch long. Weigh the juice, pulp, and boiled peel, and add broken lump sugar equal in weight to the whole, and boil for half an hour, carefully removing the scum. Then put it into pots, and when quite cold, seal them up. Some use only half bitter oranges, and the rest common sweet oranges.

JELLY OF APRICOTS.

Take the stones out of one dozen and a half of fine apricots, and boil them in the syrup, which, in this case, should be as light as possible. When boiled sufficiently to extract the flavor, and strain through a napkin, add the necessary quantity of isinglass, and finish as usual.

PRESERVING WATERMELON WITH THE PULP.

Put the melon in brine three days, then in fresh water three days, after which boil it in alum-water, repeating it several times; let it only remain until it comes to the boil each time; then keep it in fresh water a few hours. To every pound of the melon allow a pound of white sugar, and enough water to make sufficient syrup. To every six pounds of preserves allow two lemons, peeled, sliced and seeded. Flavor with ginger, and other spices.

TO PRESERVE CITRON WATERMELON.

Pare the dark green from the outside, and scrape the soft pulp from the inside of the lemon; cut in slices, boil it in alum-water till clear. Throw it into spring-water, where it may lie two or three hours, changing the water frequently. To one pound of fruit take one pound of sugar. Make a syrup of half the quantity of sugar, and boil with it all the melon until done, when it will be transparent. At the expiration of two or three days, take the jelly from it, and add the remaining half of the sugar. Boil and pour over it the melon, which will be ready for use. Season it with ginger.

Some persons follow the foregoing receipt, scalding the melons in alum-water; others soak them in pure water, and scald them by turning on the boiling syrup. If this method does not soften them enough, they should be scalded in the syrup; for as they are very hard, they should be well softened by heat. Another method is to scald them in salt water till they are soft. Then put them into spring-water as directed in the above receipt, and change the water till they are sufficiently fresh. When the melons are prepared by either of those ways, dissolve the sugar in water, using no more water than is necessary to dissolve it, and turn it, scalding hot, on the melons, and let it remain a few days. Then it will have become thin from the juice of the melons, and should be again boiled awhile and reduced to a greater degree of consistence, before pouring on the melons. It may be necessary to boil it the third time.

TO PRESERVE GOLDEN PIPPINS.

Take the rind of an orange, boil it very tender, and lay it in cold water for three days; take two dozen golden pippins, pare one-quarter of them, and boil them to a strong jelly, and run it through a jelly-bag till it is clear; take the same quantity, pare them, and take out the cores; put three pounds of loaf-sugar in a preserving-kettle, with three half-pints of spring-water. When it boils, skim it well, and put in the pippins, with the orange-rind, cut in long, thin slips; let them boil fast till the sugar is thick, and it will almost candy. Then put in three half-pints of pippin-jelly, and boil it fast till the jelly is clear. Then squeeze in the juice of a lemon, give it a boil, and put them in glass jars with the orange-peel.

APPLE MOLASSES.

There is many a good housewife who has more faith in her own experience than in the science of chemistry, that knows not the value of apple molasses; but still believes it to be the same kind of tart, smoky, worthless stuff that has from time immemorial been made by boiling down cider. It is not within my province, at this time, to attempt to convince such that there is a chemical difference, though it might easily be shown that they are almost as different as sugar and vinegar; I would, however, invite them to lay aside their cider this year, and try the plan of boiling down the juice of the apple, that has not been exposed to the air by grinding and pressing. Last autumn I placed a number of bushels of apples in two large brass kettles, with water just enough to steam them; when they had boiled soft, I turned them into a new splinter basket containing some straw, and placed on them a barrel head, and a heavy weight. The juice was caught in a tub. This was repeated until I had juice enough to fill up the kettles, when I commenced boiling it down, and attended to it strictly, frequently skimming it, till it became of the consistence of cane molasses. The native acids of the fruit imparted a peculiar flavor, otherwise it could hardly be distinguished from the syrup of the cane. It was used in my family for making sweetmeats, for sweetening pies, for dressing on puddings and griddle cakes, and a variety of other purposes. The cost of making it is very trifling, and the means are within the reach of every farmer.

APPLE BUTTER.

To make this article according to German custom, the host should, in the autumn, invite his neighbors to make up an apple-butter party. Being assembled, let three bushels of fair sweet apples be pared, quartered, and the cores removed: meanwhile let two barrels of clear new cider be boiled down to one-half; when this is done commit the prepared apples to the cider, and henceforth let the boiling go on briskly and systematically. But to accomplish the main design, the party must take turns at stirring the contents without cessation, that they do not become attached to the side of the kettle, and be burned. Let this stirring go on till the amalgamated cider and apples become as thick as hasty pudding; then throw in seasoning of pulverized allspice, when it may be considered as finished, and committed to pots for future use. This is apple butter, and will keep sweet for many years.

APPLE JELLY.

Pare, quarter, and core any quantity of fine, sound apples, cover them with water, and boil them till soft; take them out and put them into a sieve, and let all the juice drain from them into the water they were boiled in; then take the parings and some cores, cover with water and boil them; then add all the liquor of both together, and boil to a good syrup; then add one pound of sugar to one pint of syrup, and boil fifteen or twenty minutes.

PEACH JELLY.

Wipe the down well off your peaches, which should be free-stones, and not too ripe, and cut them in quarters, crack the stones, and break the kernels small; put the peaches and kernels into a covered jar, set them in boiling water, and let them boil till they are soft; strain them through a jelly-bag until all the juice is squeezed out; allow a pint of loaf-sugar to a pint of juice; put the sugar and juice into a preserving-kettle, and boil them twenty minutes, skimming very carefully; put the jelly warm into glasses, and when cold tie them up. Papers laid on the preserves, wet with brandy, help to keep them in good condition.

PEACH SWEETMEATS.

To one pound of peaches put half a pound of good brown sugar, with half a pint of water to dissolve it, first clarifying it with an egg; then boil the peaches and sugar together, skimming the egg off, which will rise on the top till it is the thickness of a jelly. If you wish to do them whole, do not peel them, but put them into boiling water and give them a boil. Then take them out, and wipe them dry. Pears are done in the same way.

TO PRESERVE GREEN FIGS.

The figs may be gathered when they have got their growth, and when they begin to turn ripe. Put them in a sieve, and pour boiling water over them to stand about an hour; then weigh the sugar, and allow pound for pound; put them in a kettle, and boil with the syrup; then take them out, and put them into dishes in the sun; boil the syrup down, put the figs back, and let them boil a short time.

TO PRESERVE TOMATOES.

Take good ripe tomatoes; peel them, and preserve them with good brown or loaf-sugar, as peaches or other fruit. If not peeled, they burst, and do not maintain the consistence so much desired by housekeepers, though they are good without peeling.

TOMATO FIGS.

Pour boiling water on the tomatoes, in order to remove the skin; then weigh, and place them in a stone jar, with as much sugar as you have tomatoes, and let them remain two days; pour off the syrup, boil and skim, until the scum ceases to rise. After this is repeated three times, they are fit to dry, if the weather is good; if not, let them remain in the syrup until drying weather. Then place on earthen plates or dishes, put them in the sun, and they will be dry in about a week; after which, pack them down in small wooden boxes, with white sugar between each layer.

HOW TO PRESERVE QUINCES WHOLE.

Take the weight of your quinces in sugar, and put a pint of water to a pound of sugar; make it into a syrup, and clarify it; then core your quinces, and pare them, and put them into your syrup, and let it boil till it be all clear; then put in three spoonsful of jelly; which must be made thus:—Over-night lay your quince kernels in water; then strain them, and put them into your quinces, and let them have but one boil afterward.

QUINCE JELLY.

Put the quinces on in cold water; boil tender, and to each quart of juice add one pound and a half of sugar. Boil about fifteen minutes, or until it jellies; it is done when it drips from the spoon.

QUINCE PRESERVES, NO. I.

Boil the quinces, (after peeling,) in enough water to cover them well; when they are perfectly soft, lay them on dishes, not touching; then take the juice in which they were boiled, strain it, and add to each pint three quarters of a pound of white sugar; boil until it is a thick syrup. Just before taking it up, put back the fruit, then pour all out together into dishes; and after it has cooled, put it up in jars, which should hold not more than one quart; cork and seal tightly.

QUINCE PRESERVES, NO. II.

Boil the quinces in clear water until they are soft, then peel and core them; take their weight in sugar; put alternately a layer of fruit and sugar in an earthen vessel, and let it remain several hours, or long enough for plenty of syrup to be formed. Add two tumblers-full of water to every two pounds of fruit; then put all together into a kettle and boil it until the fruit is about half done. Take it carefully out of the syrup, spread it on dishes, and sun it several days; then boil the syrup once more, until it is as thick as you wish it; and a few minntes before it is taken up, put the fruit in it to boil until quite soft.

TO PRESERVE STRAWBERRIES WHOLE.

Take equal weights of the fruit and refined sugar; lay the former in a large dish, and sprinkle half the sugar in fine powder over; give a gentle shake to the dish, that the sugar may touch the under sides of the fruit. Next day make a thin syrup with the remainder of the sugar, and instead of water allow one pint of red currant-juice to every pound of strawberries. In this simmer them until sufficiently jellied.

STRAWBERRY JELLY.

One pound of picked strawberries; press them lightly, and put them in four ounces of clear syrup; cover, and let them stand all night; strain through a bag on the following morning: meanwhile clarify half a pound of sugar; when nearly clarified, add to it a few drops of prepared cochineal, to give it a fine red color, after which strain it through a sieve, and add to it an ounce of clarified isinglass, the juice of two sound lemons, and afterwards the fruit. Stir the jelly gently, and put it in a mold placed on ice.

To clarify isinglass, take one ounce of the best Russia; cut it in small pieces; wash it several times in clear warm water; let it boil sufficiently in one pint of soft water, taking care to skim it well; when it is reduced to one-half, strain through a napkin into a clean vessel. The sugar and isinglass should only be lukewarm when you mix them. These remarks apply to all jellies of this kind.

PINE-APPLE JELLY.

Take a fine ripe pine-apple, cut it small, and strain the juice through a hair-sieve; then throw it into the boiling syrup, let it boil up, and, when nearly cold, strain it through a silk sieve. Add the juice of two fine lemons, and an ounce of clarified isinglass. Proceed as in strawberry jelly.

TO PRESERVE RASPBERRIES.

Pick your raspberries in a dry day, just before they are fully ripe; lay them in a dish; beat and sift their weight of fine sugar, and strew it over them. To every quart of raspberries take a quart of red currant jelly, and put to it its weight of fine sugar; boil and skim it well. Then put in your raspberries, and give them a scald. Take them off, and let them stand two hours. Then set them on again, and scald until they look clear.

RASPBERRY JAM.

Take a pint of currant-jelly, and a quart of raspberries; bruise them well together, set them over a slow fire; keep stirring all the time till it boils; let it boil gently half an hour, and stir it round very often, to keep it from sticking, and rub it through a colander; pour it into your jar, covering it tight: it will keep for a year or two, and have the full flavor of the raspberry.

TO PRESERVE GRAPES.

Get some fine grapes, not over-ripe, and pick out all the specked ones. Put them in a jar, with a quarter of a pound of sugar-candy, and fill the jar with French brandy. Tie them down close, and keep them in a dry place. You may do cherries the same way.

PRESERVED CRAB-APPLES.

Wash your fruit, cover the bottom of your preserving-kettle with grape-leaves, put in the apples, hang them over the fire, with a very little water, and cover them closely: do not allow them to boil, but let them simmer gently till they are yellow. Take them out, and spread them on a large dish to cool, pare and core them, put them again into the kettle, with fresh vine-leaves under and over them, and a very little water; hang them over the fire till they are green, not letting them boil; take them out, weigh them, and allow a pound of loaf-sugar to a pound of crab-apples, put to the sugar just water enough to dissolve; when it is all melted, put it on the fire, and boil and skim it, then put in your fruit, and boil the apples till they are quite clear and soft. Put them in jars, and pour the warm liquor over them; when cold, tie them up with brandy paper.

PRESERVED CRANBERRIES.

Wash your cranberries, weigh them, and to each pound allow a pound of loaf-sugar, dissolve the sugar in a very little water, (about half a pint of water to a pound of sugar,) and set it on the fire in a preserving kettle; boil it near ten minutes, skimming it well; then put in your cranberries and boil them slowly till they are quite soft, and of a fine color. Put them warm into your jars or glasses, and tie them up with brandy paper when cold: when opened for use, they should be tied up again immediately, as exposure to the air spoils them.

PRESERVED PINEAPPLE.

Pare your pineapples, and cut them in thin round slices; weigh the slices, and to each pound allow a pound of loaf-sugar; dissolve the sugar in a very small quantity of water, stir it, and set it over the fire in a preserving-kettle; boil it ten minutes, skimming it well; then put in it the pineapple slices, and boil them till they are clear and soft, but not till they break—about half an hour, or perhaps less time, will suffice. Let them cool in a large dish or pan before you put them into your jars, which you must do carefully, lest they break. Pour the syrup over them, and tie them up with brandy paper.

TO CLARIFY SUGAR FOR PRESERVES.

Break as much as is required in large lumps, and put a pound to a half-pint of water in a bowl, and it will dissolve better than when broken small. Set it over the fire, and add the white of an egg well beaten, let it boil up, and when ready to run over, pour a little cold water in it to give it a check; but when it rises the second time, take it off the fire, and set it by in the pan a quarter of an hour, during which the foulness will sink to the bottom, and leave a black scum on the top, which take off gently with a skimmer, and pour the syrup into a vessel very quickly from the sediment.

PREPARATIONS FOR THE SICK.

ARROW-ROOT.

Mix a dessert spoonful of arrow-root with sufficient cold water to form a soft paste; rub it till quite smooth, and add by degrees half a pint of boiling water, stirring it briskly. Boil for a minute or two, and when removed from the fire, add a tablespoonful of sherry or other white wine where wine can be allowed, with a little grated nutmeg or lemon-peel, and sugar to the taste. For young children, milk should be used instead of water, and the wine omitted: it is also more nourishing in this form for those invalids with whom milk agrees.

SAGO.

Wash an ounce of pearl sago in cold water; then boil it gently in a pint of fresh water, stirring it frequently till dissolved. It may be flavored with wine, spices and sugar as directed for arrow-root. For children, consumptives and debilitated patients, it may be made with milk instead of water. The common sago, being in larger grains, requires more time to dissolve; and is usually steeped some hours before boiling it.

TAPIOCA.

Is prepared as sago, but is more nourishing when made with milk.

BEEF TEA.

Take of lean beef, cut in shreds, one pound; water, one quart. Boil for twenty minutes, removing any scum that arises. When cold, strain it. Take half a pound of good rump-steak; cut it into thin slices, spread these into a hollow dish; sprinkle with a little salt, and pour over the whole a pint of boiling water. Cover the dish and place it near the fire for half an hour; then boil fifteen minutes, and strain through a sieve. This tea should be weakened, for invalids, with boiling water.

ESSENCE OF BEEF.

Take of lean beef, sliced, a sufficient quantity to fill the body of a porter-bottle, cork up loosely, and place it in a pot of cold water, attaching the neck, by means of a string, to the handle of the pot. Boil from one and a half to two hours, then pour off the liquid, and strain it. To this preparation may be added spices, salt, wine, brandy, &c., according to the taste of the patient, and nature of the disease.

MUTTON TEA.

Take one pound of good mutton, freed from the fat, and cut into thin slices; pour over it a pint and a half of boiling water, in the same manner as directed for beef tea; but it requires to be boiled for half an hour previous to straining. If the invalid desires the addition of barley, an ounce of clean pearl barley, washed and macerated in boiling water for an hour, may be boiled with the mutton tea, and the undissolved barley separated by straining.

CHICKEN WATER, NO. I.

Take half a chicken, divested of all fat, and break the bones; add to this, a half-gallon of water, boil for half an hour; pour off, and season with salt and pepper.

CHICKEN WATER, NO. II.

Take a small chicken, free it from the skin, and from all the fat between the muscles; divide it lengthwise into halves; remove the lungs, liver, &c., then cut it, bones and muscles, into thin slices; put these into a pan with a sufficient quantity of salt; add a quart of boiling water, cover the pan, and simmer slowly, for two hours. Strain through a fine sieve.

CHICKEN PANADA.

Take the white meat of a boiled or roasted fowl from the skin, and cut it into small pieces; pound them in a mortar, with an equal quantity of stale bread, and a sufficiency of salt, adding gradually the water in which some of the chicken has been boiled, or some beef-tea, until the whole forms a fluid paste; put this into a pan, and boil ten minutes, continually stirring.

VEGETABLE BROTH.

Take two potatoes, one carrot, one turnip, and one onion; slice and boil them in a quart of water for an hour, adding water from time to time, to keep up the original quantity; flavor with salt, and a small portion of pot-herbs, and strain. When allowable to a patient, add a small quantity of mushroom-catsup.

LIGHT BREAD SOUP.

Boil in a saucepan a pint of water, to which add an egg well beaten, two slices of bread, toasted brown, a teacup of sweet milk, a little butter, and salt and pepper to the taste.

MILK PORRIDGE.

Make a fine gruel of half grits, well boiled; strain off, and add either cold or warm milk, as preferred. Serve with toast.

FRENCH MILK PORRIDGE.

Stir some oatmeal and water together; let it stand till it gets clear, and pour off the water; then pour fresh water upon it; stir it well; let it stand till next day; strain through a fine sieve, and boil the water, adding milk while boiling. The proportion of water must be small. This, with toast, is a good breakfast for weak persons.

PANADA.

Stale bread, one ounce; cinnamon, one drachm; water, one pint; cover, and let it stand for an hour; then beat it up, and let it boil for ten minutes, adding a little grated nutmeg and sugar. Wine may be added, if desired.

PANADA.

Boil a pint of new milk; add to it half a dozen crackers, two or three spoonsful of good Sherry wine, and some grated nutmeg. The wine should not be added until the milk has been taken off the fire.

BOILED FLOUR.

Take of fine flour a pound; tie it up in a linen cloth, as tightly as possible; and after frequently dipping it into cold water, dredge the outside with flour, till a crust is formed around it whilst boiling. Boil for a long time, and permit to cool, when it will become a dry, hard mass. This is to be grated, and prepared like arrow-root. It is a good diet for children in diarrhœa, &c.

BISCUIT JELLY.

White biscuits, four ounces, to be boiled in two quarts of water, down to one quart, and strain and evaporate to one pint; add one pound of white sugar, four ounces of port-wine, and one drachm of cinnamon-water; the whole to be well mixed. It has been found useful for debility of the digestive organs.

BREAD JELLY.

Cut a French roll into slices; toast these on both sides, and boil in a quart of water until the whole forms a jelly, adding more water if required; strain and flavor. This is nutritious, and may be made more so by using broth, wholly deprived of fat, instead of water.

RICE JELLY.

This is one of the most nourishing preparations of rice for invalids. It is thus made: — Boil a quarter of a pound of rice-flour, with half a pound of loaf-sugar, in a quart of water, till the whole becomes one glutinous mass; then strain off the jelly, and let it stand to cool.

CALF'S FOOT JELLY.

Take the feet of two calves, and add to them one gallon of water, and boil down to one quart; strain, and when cold remove the fat; then add the whites of six or eight eggs, well beaten; a pint of wine; half a pound of loaf-sugar; the juice of four lemons, and mix well. Boil for a few minutes, constantly stirring; then strain through a flannel bag. The wine may be omitted, if desirable.

ICELAND MOSS.

Infuse an ounce of picked Iceland moss, for fifteen minutes, in half a pint of hot water; strain off the water, and boil the moss in a quart of fresh milk till reduced to a pint and a half. Cool it in something that will give the jelly a pretty form. The flavor is much improved by eating with fruit jelly—quince or apple—if admissible, for a patient. This dish is both nice and ornamental for a dessert or supper.

AN AGREEABLE BEVERAGE FOR A SICK PERSON.

Break up half a dozen hard biscuits or crackers in an earthen bowl; set it on a trivet with warm embers under it, and pour boiling water on the mixture until the bread is covered, and the water not too thick; leave it over the fire two or three minutes, adding sugar, allspice, and a little Sherry wine; add an egg, if desired, to be beaten in the bowl first, adding the water gradually; then the crackers, spices, &c.

TOAST WATER.

Toast thoroughly a slice of stale bread; put it into a jug, and pour over it a quart of water, which has been boiled and cooled, and in two hours pour off. A small piece of orange or lemon-peel, put into the jug with the bread, improves the flavor greatly. This forms a good drink in febrile affections.

APPLE WATER.

Slice two large apples, and pour over them a pint of boiling water; let it stand for an hour, and pour off. If necessary, sweeten with a little white sugar. It is also prepared by boiling, for an hour, ten ounces of sliced apples in two pints of water, and straining.

LEMON-PEEL WATER.

Take the rind of one lemon, and half an ounce of refined loaf-sugar; put them into a jar, and pour over them a quart of boiling water. When cold, pour off the fluid, and add a tablespoonful of lemon-juice. If wine be not improper for the invalid, a glass of Sherry may be added, instead of the lemon-juice.

BRAN TEA.

Fresh wheat bran, one pound; water, three quarts; boil down to one quart, strain, and add sugar, honey, or molasses, according to the taste of the patient.

WINE WHEY.

Boil a pint of milk, and put to it a glass of white wine; set it over the fire till it just boils again; then set it off till the curd has settled; then strain it, and sweeten to the taste.

RENNET WHEY.

Warm a pint of milk, but do not let it get too hot, or it will spoil the taste of the whey; wash the salt from a piece of rennet the size of a silver dollar, and put it in the milk; when it turns, take out the rennet, wash and put it in a cup of water, and it will do to use again to make whey. If you have rennet in a bottle of wine, two teaspoonsful of it will make a quart of whey; but if the invalid has fever, it is best to make it without wine.

MULLED WINE.

Beat together an egg, a glass of wine, and a spoonful of sugar; pour on it half a pint of water; stir all the time to keep it firm; and when you pour it in a tumbler grate a little nutmeg over it.

CHOCOLATE.

To make a cup of chocolate, grate a large teaspoonful in a mug, and pour a teacup of boiling water on it; let it stand covered by the fire a few minutes, when you can put in sugar and cream ready to drink.

BEVERAGES.

ACIDULATED RASPBERRY SYRUP.

Put six pounds of raspberries into a china or glass bowl, with a quart of water, in which has been dissolved two and a half ounces of tartaric or citric acid, and let it remain twenty-four hours. Then strain it, taking care not to bruise the fruit. To each pint of clear liquor, add one and a half pounds of pounded loaf-sugar, and stir it with a silver spoon till dissolved. Leave it for a few days; then bottle it close. A little of this syrup forms a refreshing drink in warm weather.

Acidulated strawberry syrup is made in the same way, using only two ounces of citric acid.

RASPBERRY BRANDY.

Scald the fruit in a stone jar set in a kettle of water, or on a hot hearth. When the juice will run freely, strain it without pressing. To every quart of juice allow one pound of loaf-sugar. Boil it up and skim. When quite clear, pour out; and when cold, add an equal quantity of brandy. Shake them well together, and bottle.

BLACKBERRY CORDIAL, NO. I.

To each pound of blackberries allow half a pound of sugar. After putting the blackberries and sugar (well mixed) into a large jar, cover them with good brandy. Add a few cloves, and allspice. In three weeks pour off the liquor, and bottle and cork tightly.

BLACKBERRY CORDIAL, NO. II.

Put one gallon of best brandy in a three-gallon keg; fill up with blackberries; cork and set it away for three months. Then pour off, and measure the liquor. To every quart, add a half-pound of sugar, one pint of good wine, and one pint of water. Bottle, and cork tight. It will be ready for use in six weeks.

BLACKBERRY WINE, NO. I.

To one gallon of clear blackberry juice, add one quart of water, and three pounds of white sugar. Mix well together, and put the mixture into an earthen or wooden vessel, which should be kept almost full. Skim well every twenty-four hours until it is done fermenting, which will be in about a month; then bottle, and cork tightly. Lay the bottles down on the sides, in a cool dry place. This is a receipt that can be fully relied on, if the directions are properly attended to.

BLACKBERRY WINE, NO. II.

To one quart of blackberry juice, add one pint of water, and three-quarters of a pound of sugar. Make as directed above.

BLACKBERRY SYRUP.

This syrup is said to be a specific for the summer complaint. From a teaspoonful to a wine-glass, according to the age of the patient, must be given at intervals till relieved.

How to make it: — To two quarts of juice of blackberries, add one pound of loaf-sugar, half an ounce of nutmegs, half an ounce of cinnamon pulverized, one-quarter of an ounce of cloves, one-quarter of an ounce of allspice, pulverized; boil together for a short time, and when cold add a pint of fourth-proof French brandy.

ORANGE WINE.

Of sugar twenty-three pounds, water ten gallons; boil, and clarify with the white of six eggs; pour the boiling liquor upon the parings of one hundred oranges; add the strained juice of these oranges and six ounces, or half-pint of good fresh yeast; let it work for three or four days; then strain it into a barrel; bung it up loosely. In a month add four pounds of brandy, and in three months it will be fit to drink. Wines may also be made of blackberries, and other English fruits, upon the same principles. The above are the methods generally employed; but most persons have peculiar ways of proceeding, which may indeed be varied to infinity, and so as to produce at pleasure a sweet or dry wine, the sweet not being so thoroughly fermented as the dry. The addition of brandy destroys the proper flavor of the wine, and it is better to omit it entirely (except for elder or port wine, whose flavor is so strong that it cannot well be injured), and to increase the strength by augmenting the quantity of the raisins or sugar. In general, the must for wines ought to be made of six pounds of raisins, or four pounds of sugar to the gallon, allowing for that contained in the fruit.

ORANGE SYRUP.

This syrup, so easily made, can be used so constantly with advantage, that no housekeeper should be without it. Select ripe and thin-skinned fruit, squeeze the juice through a sieve. To every pint add a pound and a half of powdered sugar. Boil it slowly, and skim as long as any scum arises. Then take it off, let it grow cold, and bottle it, taking care to secure the corks well. Two tablespoonsful of this syrup, mixed in melted butter, make an excellent sauce for plum or batter pudding. It also imparts a fine flavor to custards.

CURRANT WINE.

To each gallon of currant juice, add two gallons of water, and to each gallon of the mixture, add three and a half pounds of good brown sugar, and put into good barrels. After it has done fermenting, it should be bunged tightly for two or three weeks; then it should be racked off, and put into clean strong casks. If you wish to give it more body, add to each barrel, after it has been racked off, one gallon of good French brandy.

Gooseberry wine may also be made in the same manner.

PARSNIP WINE.

Wine made of parsnip-root approaches nearer to the Malmsley of Madeira and the Canaries than any other wine. It is made with little expense or trouble, and only requires to be kept a few years to make it agreeable to the palate as it is wholesome to the body. To every four pounds of parsnips, cleaned and quartered, put one gallon of water; boil them till they are quite tender; drain them through a sieve, but do not bruise them, as no remedy would clear them after wards. Pour the liquor into a tub, and to each gallon add three pounds of loaf-sugar, and half an ounce of crude tartar. When cooled to the temperature of 75 degrees, put in a little new yeast; let it stand four days in a warm room; then turn it. The mixture should, if possible, be fermented in a temperature of 60 degrees. September and March are the best seasons for making the wine. When the fermentation has subsided, bung down the cask, and let the wine stand at least twelve months before bottling.

GINGER WINE.

Of bruised ginger twelve pounds, water ten gallons. Boil for half an hour; add twenty-eight pounds of sugar; boil till dissolved; then cool, and put the liquor along with fourteen lemons sliced, and three pints of good French brandy; add a little yeast, and ferment; bung it up for three months, and then bottle it.

MODE OF REFINING WINE AND CIDER.

Take new, sweet skim-milk, drawn at night and skimmed the following morning, or morning's milk, skimmed at night, one pint to a quarter-cask; pour it into the liquor to be refined, the coldest weather in the winter, and stir it up thoroughly, to incorporate it completely; let it settle, and your work is done. The liquor will be pure and fine, and will have a peculiar richness imparted to it by the process.

METHEGLIN.

Of honey fifty pounds, boiling water a sufficient quantity to fill a thirty-two gallon cask; stir it well for a day or two; add yeast, and ferment. Some boil the honey in the water for an hour or two, but this hinders its due fermentation.

MEAD.

Take ten gallons of water, two gallons of honey, and a handful of raced ginger; then take two lemons, cut them in pieces, and put them into it; boil it very well; keep skimming it; let it stand all night in the same vessel you boil it in. The next morning barrel it up, with two or three spoonsful of good yeast. In two or three weeks after, you may bottle it.

HOP BEER.

For half a barrel of beer, take half a pound of hops and half a gallon of molasses. Boil the hops, adding to them a teacupful of powdered ginger, in about a pailful and a half of water; that is, a quantity sufficient to extract the virtue of the hops. When sufficiently boiled or brewed, take it up, and strain it through a sieve into a tub; add the molasses, shaking or stirring it well with a wooden ladle, that it may be thoroughly mixed. Then put it into your barrel, and fill up with water quite to the bung, observing to shake the barrel well afterwards; the bung must be left open, to allow it to work. You must be careful to keep it constantly filled up with water whenever it works over. When sufficiently worked, it may be bottled, adding a spoonful of molasses to each bottle.

SPRUCE BEER.

Put four gallons of cold water into a keg, with one head out; then, after boiling four gallons more, put that in also; add two quarts of molasses, or sweeten to your taste, and one large wine-glass of the essence of spruce, observing to stir them well together for several minutes. When about blood-warm, add one pint of good yeast, the whole being well stirred together. The top should be covered with the head, and set up carefully to work, and in two days it will be fit to bottle. By packing the bottles away in sand in the cellar, or a cool place, they will be kept from bursting, and in two or three days the wine will be ripe for drinking.

ANOTHER METHOD OF MAKING GOOD BEER.

Put two quarts of molasses into a keg, with eight gallons of cold water; stir it well, and leave one head out. Boil two ounces of allspice, two ounces of ginger, two ounces of hops, and half a pint of Indian-meal, in four quarts of water, about an hour; strain it into the keg while hot, stirring it all well together, and in twenty-four hours it will be fit for use, or to bottle.

TAR BEER FOR CONSUMPTION.

Three quarts of pure water, one quart of wheat bran, one pint of tar, and half a pint of honey. Let them simmer, over a slow fire, for three hours, in a new stone vessel; when cool, add half a pint of brewer's yeast; let it stand thirty-six hours, and it is fit for use. It must be kept in a cool place. Take a wine-glassful before each meal.

GINGER BEER, NO. I.

Infuse three ounces of bruised ginger in four gallons of boiling water, till cold. Strain through flannel. Dissolve in the liquor five pounds of loaf-sugar, and add half a pint of solid yeast, and two and a half ounces of cream of tartar. In cold weather it will be necessary to set the cask near the fire, so as to excite brisk fermentation. As soon as this subsides, rack off the clear liquor, return it into the cask, previously washed out, and allow it to work for a day or so longer. Then draw it off, and bottle it.

GINGER BEER, NO. II.

Ginger, sliced, one ounce; dried orange-peel, half an ounce; stir them in a bag, boil with a gallon of water, and strain. Add three-quarters of an ounce of tartaric acid, twenty-five drops of essence of lemon, and twenty-four ounces of loaf-sugar. When sufficiently cool, add two tablespoonsful of fresh yeast. Let the beer work for twelve hours, and bottle it.

GINGER BEER, NO. III.

Ginger, sliced, three-quarters of an ounce; essence of lemon, rubbed with twelve ounces of sugar; boiling water, half a gallon. Infuse till cold, and strain. Ferment as above, with three or four spoonsful of yeast, and bottle.

GINGER BEER, NO. IV.

Boil two and a half ounces of bruised ginger, and three pounds of sugar, in three and a half gallons of water, for twenty minutes. Put into a large pan one ounce of cream of tartar, and the juice and rind of two lemons. Pour the boiling liquor over them, and stir the whole well together. When milk-warm, add one-fourth of a pint of good ale yeast, cover it, and let it work for two or three days, skimming it frequently; then strain it through a jelly-bag into a cask; add half a pint of brandy; bung down closely, and in two or three weeks bottle in the usual way.

GINGER BEER, NO. V.

Prepare a clear decoction of infusion of ginger with sugar and lemon, as above; but, instead of fermenting it with yeast, charge it strongly with carbonic acid gas by means of a machine.

IMPERIAL POP.

Mix cream of tartar, three ounces; ginger, one ounce; white sugar, twenty-four ounces; lemon-juice, one ounce; boiling water, a gallon and a half. When cool, strain, and ferment with one ounce of yeast, and bottle.

CORN BEER.

Boil one pint of corn, until quite soft, in enough water to cover it well, and pour it into a jar. Add a quart of syrup or good molasses, a pint of sugar, a quart of dried apples, two ounces of pulverized ginger, a cup of solid yeast dissolved in a little warm water, and three gallons of water. Set it in a warm place in winter, and a cool place in summer. It will be fit for use in a day or two.

PERSIMMON BEER, NO. I.

It is made as corn beer, with the addition of the persimmons. Locusts added, also, will improve it.

PERSIMMON BEER, NO. II.

Take two-thirds of persimmons, and one-third corn meal. Mix them well together, and bake in loaves, till they are firm and hard; they should bake slowly, taking care not to burn them. Then take the loaves and throw in a clean tub, and pour on warm water enough to soften them; when all is mashed up, it will be a thin dough. Then add as much boiling water as there is dough; after stirring it sufficiently, strain it through a sieve, and put it into a keg or barrel, and in a day or two it will be fit for use.

SWEET, CLEAR CIDER THAT WILL RETAIN ITS FINE VINOUS FLAVOR, AND KEEP GOOD FOR A LONG TIME.

It is of importance in making cider, that the mill, the press, and all the materials, be sweet and clean, and the straw clear from dust. To make good cider, the fruit should be ripe, but not rotten; and when the apples are ground, if the juice is left in the pomace twenty-four hours, the cider will be richer, softer, and higher colored. If the fruit is all of the same kind, it is generally thought that the cider will be better, as the fermentation will certainly be more regular, which is of importance. The gathering and grinding of the apples, and the pressing out of the juice, are mere manual labor, performed with very little skill in the operation; but here the great art of making good cider commences: for as soon as the juice is pressed out, nature begins to work a wonderful change in it. The juice of fruit, if left to itself, will undergo three distinct fermentations, all of which change the quality and nature of this fluid. The first is the vinous; the second, the acid, which makes it hard, and prepares it for vinegar: by the third it becomes putrid. The first fermentation is the only one the juice of apples should undergo to make good cider. It is this operation that separates the juice from the filth, and leaves it a clear, sweet, vinous liquor. To preserve it in this state, is the grand secret. This is done by fumigating it with sulphur, which checks any further fermentation, and preserves it in its fine vinous state. It is to be wished that all cider-makers would make a trial of this method. It is attended with no expense, but little trouble, and will have the desired effect I would recommend that the juice, as it comes from the press, be placed in open-headed casks or vats. In this situation it is most likely to undergo a proper fermentation, and the person attending may ascertain with accuracy when this fermentation ceases. This is of great importance, and must be particularly attended to. The fermentation is attended with a hissing noise, bubbles rising to the surface and then forming a soft spongy crust over the liquid. When the crust begins to crack, and white froth appears in the cracks level with the surface of the head, the fermentation is about stopping. At this time the liquor is in a genuine, clear state, and must be drawn off immediately into casks. This is the time to fumigate it with the sulphur. To do this, take a bit of canvas or rag, about two inches broad, and twelve inches long; dip this into melted sulphur, and when a few pails of worked cider are put into the casks, set this match on fire, and hold it in the casks till it is consumed. Then bung the cask and shake it, that the liquor may incorporate with and retain the fumes. After this, fill the cask and bung it up. The cider should be racked off again the latter part of February or first of March; and if not as clear as you wish it, put isinglass into it to fine it, and stir it well. Then put the cask in a cool place, where it will not be disturbed, for the fining to settle. Cider prepared in this manner will keep for years.

KERRISON'S RECIPE FOR CIDER.

Let it be made of good, sound winter apples, in cool weather, in the month of November or December, and *let no water be mixed with it.* Put it into clean hogsheads, (whiskey hogsheads lately emptied are best), and keep it in a place invariably cool. Fermentation carries off the strength of the cider; therefore prevent it from fermenting as much as possible. When it exhibits a violent degree of fermentation, put in a half-gallon of fourth-proof rectified apple-whiskey; if this does not stop it, put in another half-gallon; the same quantity of pure French brandy will answer better where it can be had. As soon as the fermentation has subsided, and the crude particles settled down, rack it off into a clean hogshead. After this, the cider will undergo a partial fermentation; and when it has subsided, rack it off again as before. If the crude particles are allowed to remain in the hogshead, they will work up among the cider during every fermentation, and injure it. When it is being racked off, it should be allowed to run with force into a large tub, and pumped from the tub into the hogshead; this serves to break the cider, and is highly beneficial during the first and second racking. Every time it is racked, it must be bunged up tight, and the hogshead kept full; but during the fermentation, the bung should be left out. There are other methods of refining and preserving cider, which are shorter and more certain, but cannot be pursued by farmers with advantage. The above method will be found to answer all domestic purposes.

PERRY.

This is a pleasant liquor, and is made from pears, in the same manner that cider is made from apples. The pears should, in general, be ripe before they are ground. The pulp or pomace should not long remain after grinding, but should immediately be put into the press. The most crabbed and worst eating pears are said to make the best perry. The fruit may be either large or small. The more austere the pears, the better will be the liquor generally. The Taunton Squash pear (cultivated in Massachusetts) produces fruit that is held in the highest estimation in New England for perry. It is an early pear, remarkable for the tenderness of its flesh; if it drops ripe from the tree, it bursts from the fall; whence probably its name. The liquor made from it is pale, sweet, remarkably clear, and of strong body. After perry is made, it should be managed in all respects like cider; and must, if necessary, be fined by isinglass. Boiling is said by some to have a good effect on perry, changing it from a white to a flame-colored liquor, which grows better by long keeping and bottling. Good perry can scarcely be distinguished from champagne wine; is much lighter, very sparkling, lively, has a pleasanter taste; and is every way worthy of more attention, and of a more extensive manufacture than it at present receives.

LEMONADE.

Fresh lemon-juice, four ounces; fresh lemon-peel, thin, half an ounce; white sugar, four ounces; boiling water, three pints. Strain when cold.

LEMONADE IMPERIAL.

Cream of tartar, one and a half drachms; a slice of thin lemon-peel; and a lump of sugar; pour on them a quart of boiling water. Strain when cold. To be taken as a cooling drink.

COMMON LEMONADE.

Cut two lemons into slices, add two ounces of sugar, and pour on them a quart of boiling water. It is sometimes made with cold water.

MILK LEMONADE.

Dissolve half a pound of sugar in a quart of boiling water; add half a pint of fresh lemon-juice, and the same of Sherry wine; and, lastly, two-thirds of a pint of cold milk. Stir together, and strain.

ORANGEADE OR SHERBET.

Juice of four oranges; thin peel of one orange; lump-sugar, four ounces; boiling water, three pints.

CREAM NECTAR.

Take six pounds of refined sugar, four ounces of tartaric acid, two quarts of water, and when warm, add the whites of four eggs, well beaten. Be careful not to let it come to a boil, and when cool, strain it. To a teaspoonful of the above syrup, add a very small quantity of the carbonate of soda, and stir until it effervesces.

PUNCH.

To make two quarts of punch, take three fresh lemons; rub the outsides of them over with lumps of loaf-sugar, until they become quite yellow; throw the lumps into the bowl; roll the lemons well; cut them in half, and squeeze them with a proper instrument over the sugar; bruise the sugar, and continue to add fresh portions of it, mixing the lemon-pulp and juice well with it. Much of the quality of the punch depends on this. The quantity of sugar to be added should be great enough to render the mixture, without water, quite mild and palatable. Then add, gradually, a small quantity of hot water, just enough to render the syrup sufficiently thin to pass through the strainer. Mix all well together; strain it and try it; if at all sour, add more sugar. When cold, put in a little cold water, and the best French brandy and old Jamaica rum, equal quantities, adapted to the taste.

To make good punch, it is necessary to have plenty of fresh lemon-juice, an abundance of good sugar, a fair proportion of brandy and rum, and very little water.

RASPBERRY VINEGAR.

Put two pounds of raspberries in a large bowl, and pour on them two quarts of white-wine vinegar; the next day strain the liquor on two pounds of fresh raspberries; let it stand a day, and strain it into a stone jar; to each pint of the liquor put a pint of refined sugar; stir till it is dissolved, and put the jar in a sauce-pan of water, which keep boiling for an hour; skim and bottle it when cold. This is used as a refreshing drink, mixed with water. No glazed or metal vessel should be used in making it.

THE DAIRY.

PROFITS OF COW-KEEPING.

No branch of husbandry is more profitable than the keeping of cows, if properly managed. Many farmers among us are solicitous to improve their breed of cows, and some raise considerable quantities of good roots, with which to feed during the winter. This is all very good, so far; but what is the treatment of cows during the summer season, the time when all, or nearly all, the profits are obtained? Cows kept in short, dry pastures in summer, will not be profitable to their owner, however much ruta-baga, mangel-wurtzel, or carrots, have been fed out to them during the winter. I believe that the most profitable mode of keeping cows through the summer is by soiling, or feeding them with grass in the barn or yard. This may frighten some farmers, and excite the ridicule of others; but I think it will be granted, that he is the best farmer who realizes the greatest number of dollars and cents from a given quantity of land with the least amount of labor. Many farmers pride themselves on raising great crops, and one hundred bushels of Indian corn have been raised on a single acre. This is a great result; but I believe that three thousand bushels of ruta-baga may be as cheaply raised, take one year with another, as one hundred bushels of corn. Three thousand bushels of ruta-baga will give about a bushel and a half a day each to six cows throughout the whole year. It is easy enough to see that cows fed in this way will be in excellent condition, and yield immense quantities of butter and cheese.

The method of soiling, as described by Dr. Dean, was to feed cows with new-mown grass. An acre of rich ground, he says, will summer a number of cows; a little hay or grass will indeed be necessary at all times of the year; but I believe roots should be used in great abundance, and be made the chief article for feeding milch-cows throughout the year. Farmers, whose cows calve early, and who have abundance of roots, may make prodigious quantities of butter and cheese early in the spring. But how shall the farmer contrive to have a constant supply of roots throughout the summer, and until early root crops are ripe enough for use? This is a question of immense importance. Ruta-baga will keep well till July, and is it not possible that by some kind of management this root may be preserved in good condition nearly or quite through the summer? We have an account of an Englishman who buried some potatoes deep in the earth, so deep that their vegetation was prevented, and the potatoes, when kept two or three years, were of as good flavor and quality as when first ripe. It is believed that potatoes may be kept through the summer without sprouting, in a common ice-cellar. It has been contended that potatoes will not sprout where ice will not melt. Chemists pretend to describe the means which nature employs in the process of vegetation, or sprouting. Cannot chemistry tell us how some of those means can be withheld, or so managed, as to prevent, or at least retard the sprouting of vegetables? If it should be impracticable to preserve roots in good condition throughout the whole summer, I believe that if our farmers practise soiling, they will realize an ample profit by their cows: at the worst, the farmer may have a constant supply of roots for his cows, except about six weeks, from the first of July till the latter part of August; and during this short period he may supply his cows with other food. A steam-boiler is of immense advantage to every farmer who cultivates roots. Dr. Dean says that a steam-boiler is made by setting a kettle, holding twelve gallons or more, in a furnace made of brick or stone, and over this a hogshead, with one head taken out, and the other bored full of holes. With such a steam-boiler a farmer may cook the food for his milch-cows with very little fuel, and with very little labor.

Farmers in Europe and in this country have practised soiling their cattle during summer, and those who have had great experience in this mode of summering have declared it to be a much cheaper and more profitable mode than grazing. Much has been said and written of late years in regard to the great profits of root culture; but the farmer who keeps a poor breed of cattle, sheep, and swine, and whose cows in summer range in a short, dry pasture, will never realize much wealth, however great his advantages may be in other respects. The practice of soiling cows would certainly make a great saving of land, and of course it would give to farmers a large pasture for sheep. Immense quantities of manure could be made, especially by those farmers who are not afraid of a little labor in hauling muck, loam, and other materials calculated to absorb the urine of animals, which is most commonly entirely lost.

A GOOD STEAM-BOILER.

The Editor of the Nashville Agriculturist says:— "After studying some time how to construct a cheap and convenient boiler, sufficient to cook food for the cattle on my small farm, I have at length succeeded. I purchased a kettle holding sixty gallons, and with the labor of two hands for one day, constructed a furnace of rough lime-stone. I then made a box of rough plank, three feet square at the bottom, and high enough to hold about ten bushels; the box was perforated with many holes by the use of a five-quarter auger. The bottom of the box is made with plank six feet long, to afford projections to lift it on and off the kettle.

"When the cooking process is going on, the top of the box is covered with a piece of carpet, or a close-fitting plank cover to keep in the steam. In using this apparatus, a bushel or two of corn or roots may be put in the kettle, and the box filled with cut oats, corn-stalks, turnip-tops, beets, potatoes, or any thing else that grows on the farm, and the whole may be thoroughly cooked in an hour or two."

FEEDING COWS IN WINTER.

An equal quantity of shelled corn, peas, and pumpkins, boiled together until done, and cooled before being given to the cows. Stock peas and corn alone, would also be good food; or peas and meal, with or without pumpkins, are excellent. They should be well sheltered in inclement weather, and well curried and rubbed every morning and evening during the year.

ANOTHER WAY TO FEED COWS.

Boil equal quantities of corn or corn meal and carrots; or wheat bran, peas, and corn. Clean slops from the kitchen are also good.

HOW TO MILK.

Give the cow an easy and pleasant place to stand. Approach her gently. Have a good stool, and sit on it, if the cow will let you while milking. Commence very gently, especially if the cow is sensitive, or her udder or her teats are sore. When you have fairly begun, milk with a regular easy motion, and as fast as you can, without fatigue, till you are done. Milk very clean. If you have too many cows for one person to milk, it is much better to have the same person always milk the same cows. A cow is better contented, and will give more milk, if she is always milked by the same person.

TO KEEP MILK SWEET.

Be careful to have your milk-vessels well scalded and sunned several hours before using them. As soon as your milk is strained, set it in a tin or porcelain vessel over a fire until it is quite hot, then pour it into your milk-vessels, which should not be more than eight inches deep, with covers to fit tight. The cream rises much better in shallow vessels; and it should be skimmed off in twenty-four hours, and churned immediately in warm weather; in cold weather, it will be necessary to let it remain longer; it will require a longer time for the cream to become acid. It is best to put it near a fire in cold weather.

MAKING BUTTER.

Salt and work the butter when it comes from the churn; work again the next day without cold water in any of the processes, and then pack tight in tubs lined with bags, previously saturated with beeswax, and cover on the top with clean pickle. The great requisites in making and preserving good butter are; 1st. That everything should be cleanly in the whole process. 2nd. That milk should be kept at a proper temperature, say from 45° to 55°, while the cream is separating. 3rd. That the cream should be taken off and churned before its quality is impaired. 4th. That its temperature should be from 55° to 65° when put into the churn, and the churning should be moderate and uniform. 5th. That salt, of the best quality (say alum salt made fine,) in sufficient quantity to suit the palate, should be blended with it in the first working, and the buttermilk completely got out by the butter-ladle. 6th. That the working of the butter should be repeated at the end of twenty-four hours, when the salt has become completely dissolved, and all the liquid extracted. 7th. That it should be packed without more salt to make it weigh, in stone jars, in wooden firkins or tubs, such as will not impart to it any taint or bad flavor, and in such a manner as will totally exclude the atmosphere. Butter made in this way will be of fine flavor; and, by observing the directions, and keeping it in a temperature below 70°, will retain its sweetness a long time. Water mixed either with the milk, the cream, or the butter, and especially soft water, adds nothing to, but materially detracts from its richness of flavor. Milk skimmed at three several times, will give three qualities of butter; that taken off first being the richest and most valuable.

When there is a difficulty of obtaining good butter quick in churning, it is said, by adding a tablespoonful of good vinegar to four gallons of cream it may be obtained in a few minutes.

PATENT BUTTER.

A Prussian nobleman has received from the Emperor letters patent, as a reward for discovering a new method of making butter, which may be of importance to dairy-women in this country. The process consists in boiling, or rather simmering the milk, for the space of fifteen minutes, in its sweet state, taking care not to burn it; and then churning it in the usual manner. It is said no difficulty ever occurs in making butter immediately, and of a quality far superior to that made from milk which has undergone vinous fermentation. Butter made in this manner is also said to preserve its flavor and sweetness much longer than butter made in the ordinary manner. The milk likewise being left sweet, is considered of nearly the same value as before churning, and far more healthy on account of its having the animalculæ, or whatever else it may have contained, destroyed. The ease with which the experiment may be made, should induce all to give it a fair trial.

SALTING BUTTER.

It is not unfrequently that we hear complaints, which, we have no doubt, are well founded, that much of the butter for sale in our market is strongly rancid and unfit for use. But where lies the fault? Our dairy-women are not altogether chargeable with the evil; many of them know their duty and do it faithfully, as far as the manufacture of the article is concerned. When it is first made, it is pure and sweet, and they do all in their power to preserve it in that state; but, in spite of all their efforts, after it has remained a short time it will become strong, bitter, and disagreeable. From our own experience we are induced to believe, that the greatest part of the fault is in the salt which is used in it. We are never able to preserve butter in its purity, for any length of time, salted with the Liverpool salt; while the butter made in the same way, and salted with the ground rock-salt, has been kept a year, retaining the same sweet and pleasant flavor it possessed when first taken from the churn. That the fine Liverpool salt is not fit to be used to preserve meat or butter is a fact not so generally known as it should be; its convenience for use, and white texture, induce people to buy it. But if, instead of this, they would purchase the ground rock-salt, notwithstanding they would have to pay a higher price, they would be gainers in the end. Dr. Mitchell, of New York, analyzed the Liverpool salt, and, after thoroughly examining its properties, he condemns the use for any purpose whatever, and says the loss of property consequent upon the employment of this salt is prodigious. Experience, year after year, has proved it to be incapable of preserving our beef from corruption. Often has this important article of food been found to be tainted the very autumn in which it has been packed in barrels; besides the sacrifice of property, we find that the employment of Liverpool salt, in the packing of beef and pork, leaves them liable to corrupt; and the consequences of this corruption are pestilential exhalations, stirring up yellow fever and other malignant distempers in the neighborhoods, cities, and vessels where the bodies of those slaughtered animals are deposited.

The butter of the New York market has also been rendered worse, if not absolutely spoiled, by the same kind of salt. Beguiled by its fine and showy exterior, the citizens have used it extensively in our country, famous for grazing and dairies. In many cases it has supplanted the old-fashioned coarse or sun-made salt. Whenever the substitution has been made, it has been with a pernicious effect. The butter so salted does not keep so well, and loses its agreeable odor. The difference between butter put up with this salt, and with natural crystallized salt, is so great, that our wholesale and retail grocers can distinguish it at once by the smell, on piercing or opening a firkin. The sweet flavor and nice odor which pure sea salt gives is altogether wanting in that which we get from Liverpool. The fault of Liverpool salt, and of all other salt obtained from sea-water by force of fire or by boiling, is its admixture with foreign ingredients, known by the technical names of slack and bittern. These usually adhere to sea salt in considerable quantities. They have no antiseptic virtues, but possess a directly contrary effect. Sea salt, formed by natural evaporation and crystallization, has very little mixture with these foul and foreign ingredients.

PACKING BUTTER.

Take a stone pot, or jar, that will hold thirty or forty pounds; clean it thoroughly, and wash it in cold, strong brine. Take new, sweet butter, well made and free from buttermilk; work it well, and put a layer of it, a few inches in thickness, in the jar; beat it down solid with a wooden beater, turning off the milk that will escape occasionally; then repeat the process, until the pot is filled within an inch and a half of the top with butter thoroughly pounded down.; on the top of this pour one inch of clear brine, made by dissolving salt in warm water, and put on when cold; cork the jar tight, and tie over a cloth or piece of buckskin; keep the jar at a low temperature, and the butter will keep good and sweet for an indefinite length of time, only needing examining occasionally to see that it is covered with the brine, and renewing it if necessary.

MEDICAL RECEIPTS.

BATHING.

If every morning, and, when the heat is oppressive, every evening, the whole surface of the body were bathed in water, fresh from the pump or well, with a sponge, or rubbed well with the hands, so that the pores are cleansed, and the skin rubbed dry, the population of the city and country in which so excellent a custom prevailed would be remarkable for health, let the climate be as it might. A strong nerve, and solidity of flesh, would be gained by the process, which would set the heat of summer, and the cold of winter, at defiance. Thousands of diseases which now haunt our crowded communities would become obsolete. Thirst would not be so much excited, and the temptation to deluge the stomach with fluids would be removed. Perhaps, among all the evil practices which produce disease and weakness, none is more injurious, or prevalent, than the habit of impairing digestion by filling the stomach with fluids. As remarked before, a healthy state of the skin would diminish the practice by taking away the inducement. Upon mothers, nurses, and others who have charge of children, the frequent lavations of their little charge cannot be too much urged. Physicians tell us that two-thirds of the infantile diseases which occur, owe their origin and their aggravation to a neglect of cleanliness. It is not enough that a child's face is clean; the whole body should be so frequently washed, that the skin may perform the functions for which nature intended and curiously constructed it.

The annexed rules (which experience has established, and physiology approved) are submitted for the benefit of bathers:—

1. Bathe one hour before breakfast, or, what is much better, one hour before dinner.

3. Never take the cold bath when the temperature of the body is below the natural standard.

4. To prepare the tepid bath, which is the best in a warm climate, the rule should be this:—Bring the water to that temperature which feels neither hot nor cold to the arm, or some part of the body usually covered, and, after entering the bath, raise its heat to that point which imparts the most agreeable feeling.

5. We should take exercise before and after the warm bath; the importance of this is every day evinced where bathing is practised.

6. After leaving the water, the body should be briskly wiped with a coarse towel, and immediately covered with sufficient clothing to excite or preserve the healthy temperature.

7. We should never remain long in the water; from ten to fifteen minutes is sufficient.

8. Every second or third day is often enough to take the bath.

THE TIME REQUIRED TO DIGEST DIFFERENT ARTICLES OF FOOD.

	Hours.	Min.
Boiled rice	1	00
Sago, tapioca, barley, and boiled milk	2	15
Tripe and pigs' feet	1	00
Fowls, and beeves' liver	2	30
Hard eggs	3	30
Soft eggs	3	00
Custard	2	45
Trout, boiled or fried	1	30
Other fresh fish	3	00
Beef, rare or roasted	3	00
Dry, roasted	3	30
Salt beef, with mustard	2	30
Pickled pork	4	30
Raw pork	3	00
Roasted pork, fat and lean	5	15
Fried pork	4	15
Stewed pork	3	00
Mutton broiled	3	00
Mutton boiled	3	00
Veal fried	4	30
Fowls boiled	4	00
Fowls roasted	4	00
Ducks roasted	4	00
Wild ducks roasted	4	30
Suet, beef fresh, boiled	5	00
Suet, mutton, boiled	4	30
Butter melted	3	30
Mutton, fresh	3	15
Veal, fresh, broiled	4	00
Wheat bread, fresh baked	3	30
Corn bread	3	15

	Hours.	Min.
Sponge cake	2	30
Succatash	3	45
Apple dumplings	3	00
Apples, sour and mellow	2	00
Apples, sweet and mellow	1	30
Parsnips boiled	2	30
Potatoes boiled	3	30
Potatoes roasted	2	30
Raw cabbage	2	30
Raw, with vinegar	2	00
Cabbage boiled	4	30
Cheese, old	3	30
Soup beef, vegetables, and bread	4	00
Barley soup	1	30
Chicken soup	3	00
Oyster soup	3	30
Green corn and beans	3	45
Hash, meat, and vegetables	2	30
Sausage, fresh broiled	3	20
Codfish, boiled	2	00
Oysters, fresh and raw	2	55
Oysters roasted	3	15
Oysters stewed	3	30
Salmon, salted and boiled	4	00

METHOD OF RESTORING LIFE TO THE APPARENTLY DROWNED,

Recommended by the Royal Humane Society of England, instituted in 1774.

Avoid all rough usage. Do not hold up the body by the feet, nor roll it on casks, nor rub it with salt, or spirits, or apply tobacco. Lose not a moment in carrying the body to the nearest house, with the hands and shoulders raised. Place it in a warm room, if the weather is cold. Preserve silence, and positively admit no more than three intelligent persons. Let the body be instantly stripped, dried, and wrapped in hot blankets, which are frequently to be renewed. Keep the mouth, nostrils, and throat free and clean. Apply warm substances to the back, spine, pit of the stomach, armpits, and soles of the feet. Rub the body with heated flannel, or cotton, or warm hands. Attempt to restore breathing by gently blowing with a bellows in one nostril, closing the mouth and other nostril. Press down the breast carefully with both hands, and then let it rise again, and thus imitate natural breathing. Keep up the application of heat; continue the rubbing; increase it when life appears, and then give a teaspoonful of warm water, or very weak brandy and water, or wine and water. Persevere for six hours. Send quickly for medical assistance.

REMEDY IN CASE OF SWALLOWING PINS, FISH OR OTHER SHARP BONES.

Administer four grains of tartar emetic in warm water, and let the patient drink the white from six eggs, which, coagulating upon the stomach before the tartar operates, envelopes the piece or bone, and it is brought up. A person who had swallowed several pins was made to throw up the whole by the above method.

TO STOP BLOOD.

It has been found that soot applied to a fresh wound will not only stop the bleeding, but ease the pain.

A STYPTIC, WHICH WILL STOP THE BLEEDING OF THE LARGEST VESSELS.

Scrape fine two drachms of castile soap, and dissolve it in two ounces of brandy, or other common spirits. Mix well with it one drachm of potash, and keep it in a close phial. When applied, warm it, and dip pledgets of lint, and the blood will suddenly coagulate some distance within the vessel. For deep wounds and amputated limbs, repeated applications may be necessary.

BLEEDING AT THE NOSE.

Bathe the nose in vinegar.

TO CLEANSE THE TEETH, AND IMPROVE THE BREATH.

To four ounces of fresh prepared lime-water add one drachm of Peruvian bark, and wash the teeth with the water in the morning before breakfast, and after supper. It will effectually destroy the tartar on the teeth, and remove the offensive smell arising from those decayed.

FROST BITTEN.

Bathe the affected parts in warm beef pickle.

BURDON'S EXCELLENT OINTMENT.

Yellow resin, the size of a hen's egg, to be melted in an earthen-pot over a slow fire, to which, add the same quantity of beeswax; when melted, add half a pound of hog's lard, and, when that is dissolved, add two ounces of honey, and half a pound of common turpentine, and keep gently boiling a few minutes, stirring all the time; take it off the fire, and when it has cooled a little, stir into it two ounces of verdigris, finely powdered; then give the whole a few minutes gentle boiling, and pour through a sieve for use. Nothing takes fire out of a burn or scald in human flesh so soon as this ointment. It is equally good for cuts and bruises, and putrefying sores, and might be denominated, with propriety, the universal remedy.

OPODELDOC.

Take of Castile soap, powdered, three ounces; camphor, one ounce; brandy, one pint. Dissolve the soap in the spirits, by the fire, then add the camphor.

CURE FOR THE STING OF A WASP OR BEE.

Apply an onion, by binding it to the part affected, which is stated to be a certain cure.

ANOTHER.

Bind on the place a thick plaster of common salt moistened: it will soon extract the venom.

CURE FOR A SNAKE OR SPIDER BITE.

Take the yolk of an egg, stir with it as much salt as will make it thick enough not to run. Spread a plaster, and apply it to the wound.

CURE FOR THE BITE OF THE VIPER OR RATTLESNAKE, NO. I.

In some parts of the world many persons procure their livelihood by catching vipers. They are employed by chemists, apothecaries, &c. I remember some years ago, while in England, to have read in the Royal Society, in London, a curious circumstance of one of these viper-catchers. A member of the society had casually received information that a man engaged in this business was frequently bitten, and that he cured himself with sweet-oil. After considerable inquiry, the viper-catcher was found, and the questions asked whether he cured himself by the oil, and whether he was willing to satisfy a number of gentlemen of the fact. The man answered in the affirmative to both questions. Accordingly a very numerous meeting of the Royal Society was convened, including a considerable number of the nobility. The viper-catcher attended, accompanied by his wife and a large viper; and laying his arm naked to the shoulder, suffered the irritated reptile to strike, which it did very forcibly. His wife permitted the poison to operate, till her husband's head, face, and tongue, were greatly swollen, his arm and face turned very black, and his senses much affected, when she applied the oil by pouring a small quantity down his throat, and bathing the part bitten. The man gradually recovered. The circumstance being strongly impressed upon my mind, and knowing the poison of an English viper is considered in that country the most venomous in nature, determined me to try its power in the bite of a rattlesnake, the first opportunity that should offer in the district that I reside in. Afterward I was travelling through Pendleton, South Carolina, and met a man who inquired of me if I could assist to relieve the pain of a person who had been bitten by a large rattlesnake. Although sorry for the man's misfortune, I rejoiced at the opportunity thus offered to ascertain fully the properties of sweet-oil as an antidote to this deadly poison. Having a phial of this oil in my pocket, I hastened to the suffering creature, and on seeing him, his appearance struck me as the most frightful I had ever beheld. His head and face were extremely swollen, and the latter black; his tongue proportionably enlarged, and extending out of his mouth; his eyes appeared as if they would shoot from their sockets, and his senses gave every appearance of death. He had been bitten on the side of the foot. I immediately, but with great difficulty, poured down his throat two tablespoonsful of the oil. Its effects were almost instantaneous, and exceedingly powerful in counteracting the poison, as appeared by the strong, though quick convulsions which followed. In about thirty minutes it operated strongly, both as an emetic and cathartic, after which the swelling of the head, face, &c., gradually abated, and the tongue began to assume its place. In two hours he was so far recovered as to articulate, and from that time recovered fast till he got perfectly over it. The oil inwardly taken, and externally applied, did not exceed seven spoonsful. The number of cases of the like nature in twelve years has been considerable to which sweet oil has proved itself to be peculiarly adapted, and fully adequate to the worst of cases, if timely applied. It is a remedy which every person can command (when others cannot be procured), and ought not to be without. Indeed, many cautious persons have carried a small phial of oil constantly about them. It has also been used with equal success, when horses, cattle, dogs, &c., have been bitten. One case I am credibly informed, occurred where the oil succeeded when given to a woman who had been bitten by a small dog, and who exhibited strong symptoms of hydrophobia.

CURE FOR THE BITE OF THE VIPER OR RATTLESNAKE, NO. II.

A weed with a smooth leaf, and bulbous, milky root, known by the name of "Lion's tongue," when applied in a proper manner, is a good remedy. Mode of application: take a handful of the roots, wash clean, and boil in sweet milk. Let the patient drink occasionally of the milk thus boiled, and apply the root as a poultice to the wound, keeping it moist with the milk.

CURE FOR THE BITE OF THE VIPER OR RATTLESNAKE, NO. III.

A simple and convenient remedy is alum. A piece the size of a hickory-nut, dissolved in water and drunk, or chewed and swallowed, is sufficient. It has been tried many times on men and dogs, and they have invariably recovered.

TO CURE THE BITE OF A RATTLESNAKE, OR MAD DOG.

It is said that a strong decoction of the boiled bark of the root of the black-ash will cure the bite of a rattlesnake, or mad dog. Take a wine-glass full three times a day, for nine days.

CURE FOR HYDROPHOBIA, NO. I.

Take two ounces of the fresh leaves of the tree-box; two ounces of the fresh leaves of rue; one half-ounce of sage; chop these fine, and boil in a pint of water, down to a half-pint; strain carefully, and press out the liquor very firmly. Put back the ingredients again, and add a pint of milk, and boil down again to half a pint, and strain as before; then mix both liquors together, of which, give one-third part, each subsequent morning, fasting. As it possesses no power to relieve the disease itself, but is given merely as a preventive, any time between the reception of the bite and the first appearance of the symptoms is the proper period for administering it.

CURE FOR HYDROPHOBIA, NO. II.

For the bite of a mad dog, let the person bit, immediately drink a pint of good white-wine vinegar; repeat this three mornings, fasting, and wash the part well with vinegar at the fire; then take a large spoonful of the juice of rue three mornings, fasting; after the vinegar, before you take the rue, let about eight ounces of blood be taken away.

ANTIDOTE FOR POISON BY ARSENIC.

Salad or olive oil taken warm, and repeated occasionally, will infallibly prevent any bad consequences, if the arsenic has not been taken very long before. It is the true antidote for arsenic, and should immediately be made use of, as soon as it is discovered that any person has swallowed it by mistake or otherwise. A gentle vomit given just after taking it, and then repeatedly drinking very fat mutton broth, will effectually cure it; by this method, Sir Hans Sloane saved the life of a young man, who, at his house at Chelsea, had drunk a quantity of milk, into which arsenic had been put to poison rats.

ONIONS, AN ANTIDOTE FOR POISON.

I once knew a man who took eleven grains of arsenic in warm tea, in order to kill himself. Three physicians exerted their skill to save him, but to no purpose. By their consent, another person proposed onions, which were immediately applied to his stomach, arm-pits, wrists, and all the tender parts of his body. Though he was much swelled, he immediately began to recover, and the next day went to his work. It appeared like a miracle to all who witnessed it.

A REMEDY FOR ARSENIC.

Tobacco is said to be an infallible preventive against the fatal effects of arsenic, when taken into the stomach. In several instances where tobacco-juice was swallowed after taking arsenic, no sickness resulted from the use of the tobacco, and not the least harm from the arsenic.

ANTIDOTES FOR VARIOUS POISONS.

For Belladonna, or Nightshade.

Give emetics, and then strong acids, such as vinegar or lemon-juice and water.

Oxalic Acid.

This acid is sometimes mistaken for Epsom salts. Give magnesia, soap and water, or chalk and water, freely; then administer emetics.

Tartar Emetic.

Give tea made of Peruvian bark, galls, or white oak bark, in large quantities.

Saltpetre.

Give an emetic, then flaxseed tea, or milk and water in large quantities.

Corrosive Sublimate.

Give soap and water, or whites of eggs.

REMARKS.

In most cases of poisoning, emetics produce a good effect. An excellent emetic, and one most always at hand, is common mustard.

A spoonful of mustard flour, mixed in warm water, should be given every five or ten minutes, until the patient vomits freely. Warm, soothing drinks are beneficial, and should be administered, if medical aid cannot be immediately obtained. These drinks may be flaxseed or slippery elm tea, or chalk-water.

For external poisoning, from such plants as sumac, dogwood, &c., a solution of an ounce of copperas in a pint of water may be used to bathe the affected part.

SYMPTOMS ATTENDING SUCH AS ARE POISONED.

A pain in the breast, difficulty of breathing, a load at the pit of the stomach, an irregular pulse, burning and violent pains of the viscera above and below the navel; restlessness at night; sometimes wandering pains over the whole body; a retching inclination to vomit; profuse sweats (which prove always serviceable); slimy stools, both when costive and loose; the face of a pale yellow color; sometimes a pain and inflammation of the throat; the appetite is generally weak. Those who have been long poisoned, are generally very feeble and weak in their limbs; the whole skin peels, and the hair falls off.

Cases of poison frequently occur, especially in the southern part of the United States, from coming in contact with a common "plant," called "Poison Oak." The skin once affected, almost invariably breaks out at the same period of the year, for many years in succession.

We give below a prescription which cured every case in which it has been used.

Compound syrup of sarsaparilla, one pint.
Iodid of potash, one drachm.
Corrosive sublimate, two grains.

First rub the corrosive sublimate and potash together in a little alcohol. After it completely dissolves, add the syrup gradually, while you continue the rubbing, until the whole be thoroughly mixed. Bottle it, and take for a dose one hour before, or three hours after each meal, one tablespoonful; keep the bowels gently open, and live lightly. The parts affected should, in addition, be thoroughly washed three or four times a day with tincture of lobelia.

FOR BURN, SCALD AND CHILBLAINS.

Apply strong alum water; keep it ready prepared in a bottle. Apply it by wetting a cloth-compress, and renew it until the inflamation is removed.

REMEDY FOR BURNS.

For fourteen years I have prescribed the following remedy, and think that no disease or injury to the human system has a more certain one than this is for the most distressing of all injuries, that of scalds and burns. The first knowledge I had of it was the almost miraculous cure of a little boy who fell into a half-hogshead of boiling water, prepared for scalding hogs. The entire person and limbs of the boy passed under the scalding water up to the chin, so as to scald his whole neck. On removing his clothes, nearly all the skin followed from his neck, hands, arms, chest, back, abdomen, and almost every bit of skin from his lower extremities. In this deplorable condition, literally flayed alive with scalding water, the remedy was applied, as a momentary application, until medical help should arrive. Two eminent physicians soon came, and on hearing of the extent of the scald, pronounced it a certainly fatal case, and directed the boy to remain with the remedy over him until he should die. In six weeks he was restored quite well, with scarcely a scar on any part of his person or limbs.

The remedy is the more valuable from the fact, that, under almost all circumstances, it may be obtained. It is as follows: — Take soot from a chimney where wood is burned, rub it fine, and mix one part of soot with three parts or nearly so of hogs' lard, fresh butter, or any kind of animal grease that is not salted. Spread this on linen, or muslin, or any cotton, for easier or more perfect application.

In case of very extensive burns or scalds the cloth should be torn into strips of suitable size and shape, before putting over the scald. Let the remedy be freely and fully applied, so as perfectly to cover all the burned parts. No other measure is required until the patient is well, except to renew, at proper intervals, applications of the soot and lard. In steamboat explosions this remedy can in nearly all cases be at once applied; and if resorted to at once, in such emergencies, many valuable lives would doubtless be saved, and a vast amount of suffering alleviated.

REMEDY FOR TOOTH-ACHE.

A remedy for this most painful affliction, which has succeeded in ninety-five cases out of a hundred, is alum reduced to an impalpable powder two drachms, nitrous spirit of ether seven drachms, mixed and applied to the tooth.

ANOTHER.

Make a solution of camphor and pulverized cayenne pepper: dip in this a small quantity of raw cotton, and apply it to the affected tooth, and it will give instant relief. To prevent the composition from getting to the throat, lay a bit of rag over it for a few moments.

CURE FOR GANGRENE.

In a fight between a party of Indians, and a small party of Americans, in Texas, a leg of one of the party was shattered during the action by a musket-ball, and mortified; and having no surgical instruments, nor medicine of any kind, some live-oak bark was boiled very strong, and thickened with powdered charcoal and Indian-meal, and a poultice of it tied round his leg, over which was sewed a Buffalo skin, and the party travelled along five days without looking at it. When it was opened, the mortified parts had all dropped off, and it was in a fair way for healing, which it finally did.

TO PREVENT THE DISCOLORING OF THE SKIN BY A BRUISE.

Immediately rub on lamp-oil with the hand, or apply cloths dipped in hot water until the bruised blood disappears.

TO STOP VOMITING.

Drink very warm water, or, apply cloths wet with brandy, warm to the chest. Mustard-plasters are also excellent.

TO CURE SEED WARTS.

Apply a little aquafortis to their tops two or three times a day for a short time.

A CURE FOR CORNS.

Dip a small piece of cotton in lamp or whale oil, apply it to the corn, and wrap a bandage round it; repeat this for six or eight days, when the corn becomes soft, and is easily removed. The experiment has been tried with success.

CURE FOR HEARTBURN.

Drink a teacupful of camomile tea, or a small quantity of chalk, scraped into a glass of water: or a small teaspoonful of magnesia in a glass of water.

AN EXCELLENT PILL FOR INDIGESTION. INACTIVE STATE OF THE LIVER. A STATE OF THINGS KNOWN BY THE NAME OF DYSPEPSIA.

Take blue mass, twenty-four grains; quinine, twenty-four grains; rhubarb, twenty-four grains. Mix with compound syrup of rhubarb, or honey, or syrup, and divide into twenty-four pills; dose, one pill at bed-time.

REMEDY FOR INDIGESTION.

Boil half a pint of white wheat three hours in a quart of water, or a little more if necessary. Drink half a pint of the liquid two or three times a week.

CURE FOR CONSTIPATION.

Take a new-laid egg, raw; add to it three times its bulk of cold water; beat for thirty minutes, and take on an empty stomach. It may be taken twice a day; the first time early in the morning, and the second time between eleven and twelve o'clock; increase the quantity to three eggs in the course of ten days. Said to be good for the lungs.

FOR CONSTIPATION.

Take nice rye in the grain; soak and boil it moderately till perfectly tender, and season it with molasses, sugar, or honey. Make it a standing dish for breakfast. It may be eaten oftener if necessary.

AN INFALLIBLE REMEDY FOR A COLD.

As soon as there are symptoms of a cold, bathe in a tub of cold water for a minute or two; then rub the skin well with a coarse towel, until it is perfectly dry, and a warm glow is created.

If it is not convenient to bathe in a tub, sponging well, and using friction afterwards, often answers the purpose as well. This simple remedy would, in many cases, save much suffering, and even life, if attended to at the commencement of a cold.

REMEDY FOR COLDS.

Take a large teaspoonful of flaxseed, with half a stick of liquorice, and a quarter of a pound of sun raisins; put them into two quarts of soft water, and let it simmer over a slow fire till it is reduced to one; then add to it a quarter of a pound of brown sugar, and a tablespoonful of white wine vinegar, or lemon-juice.

The vinegar should be added only to that quantity you are going to take; for if it be put into the whole, it is liable in a little time to grow flat. Drink half a pint at going to bed, and take a little when the cough is troublesome.

This receipt generally cures the worst of colds in two or three days. It is a balsam cordial for the lungs, without the opening qualities which endanger fresh colds on going out. It has been known to cure colds that have almost been settled into consumptions, in less than three weeks.

CURE FOR INFLUENZA.

Take equal parts of good vinegar and water: to a teacupful of this mixture add one teaspoonful of Cayenne; sweeten with honey or sugar. Dose: a tablespoonful at going to bed, and one during the night, if the cough be troublesome.

A SIMPLE REMEDY FOR A COUGH.

Sweet spirits of nitre, syrup of squills, and paregoric, each one ounce. Mix, and give a teaspoonful for a dose, and repeat at short intervals, until the cough is relieved.

CURE FOR A COUGH.

Take equal parts of the moss that grows on white oak, white maple, and white ash trees. Mix, and make a strong tea; sweeten, and drink freely.

CURE FOR WHOOPING-COUGH, NO. I.

Take equal parts of sweet-oil, honey, and vinegar, and simmer together over a fire. Dose: a teaspoonful, or more, if necessary.

CURE FOR WHOOPING-COUGH, NO. II.

Take a good handful of dried colt's-foot leaves, cut them small, and boil them in a pint of water, till half a pint is boiled away; then take it off the fire, and when it is almost cold, strain it through a cloth, squeezing the herb as dry as you can; and then throw it away, and dissolve in the liquor an ounce of sugar-candy, finely powdered; and then give the child (if it be about three or four years old, and so in proportion) one spoonful of it, cold or warm as the seasons prove, three or four times a day, or oftener if the fits of coughing come frequently, till well, which will be in a few days.

CURE FOR THE ASTHMA, NO. I.

One ounce pulverized columbo, one ounce lobelia herb, one ounce hira-picra, one ounce skunk cabbage, one ounce assafœtida, one ounce ginger, one ounce elecampane, one ounce nerve-powder, one ounce rhubarb, one ounce hoarhound, and two quarts of good gin. One wine-glassful twice a day.

CURE FOR THE ASTHMA, NO. II.

Milk of gum ammoniac, three ounces; syrup of squills, two ounces; wine of ipecac, one ounce; tincture of lobelia, half an ounce. Dose: a teaspoonful four or five times a day.

REMEDY FOR CROUP, NO. I.

Syrup of ipecac, syrup of squills, comp., of each one ounce; tincture of assafœtida, half an ounce. Mix. Dose, for a child from two to four years old, commence with half a teaspoonful; increase the dose, and repeat, until free vomiting ensues. At the same time this medicine is being given, place the child in a tub of water as warm as it can be borne. When the child is taken from the bath, have ready a hot mush poultice covered with mustard, which you will apply to its throat and breast. Should the above not relieve, give five or six grains of calomel, and cup freely over the upper part of the chest.

REMEDY FOR CROUP, NO. II.

Cut onions into thin slices; between and over them put brown sugar. When the sugar is dissolved, a teaspoonful will frequently produce immediate relief.

Cause of Croup in Infants:—Eberle, in his excellent work on the diseases of children, says that the mode of dressing infants with their necks and upper part of the breast bare, cannot fail to render them subject to the influence of cold, and its dangerous consequences. In the country, especially among the Germans, who are in the habit of clothing their children in such a manner as to leave no part of the breast and lower portion of the neck exposed, croup is an exceeding rare disease. Whereas in cities, or among people who adopt the modes of dress common in cities, this frightful disease is, in proportion to the population, vastly more frequent.

REMEDY FOR CROUP, NO. III.

If a child is taken with the croup, instantly apply cold water, ice-water if possible, suddenly and freely to the neck and chest with a sponge; the breathing will almost instantly be relieved. So soon as possible, let the sufferer drink as much as it can, then wipe it dry, cover it up warm, and soon a quiet slumber will relieve the parent's anxiety.

PUTRID SORE THROAT.

Take one ounce of Jesuit's bark, one ounce of gum myrrh; boil both in two quarts of water, over a gentle fire; strain it, and give a tablespoonful every hour, after gargling with sage, honey, and saltpetre.

FOR SORE THROAT, AND DIFFICULTY OF BREATHING.

Mix a half-teaspoonful of camphor with a wine-glass of brandy; drop a little on a lump of sugar, and let a lump melt in the mouth hourly. The third or fourth generally enables the patient to swallow with ease.

THE PILES.

Take a lump of strong British alum, about two inches in length, which smooth down with a knife to the thickness of three-quarters of an inch. Apply this, first wetting it with cold water, every morning and evening for five or seven days.

RHEUMATIC OIL, NO. I.

Two ounces of sweet-oil, one ounce of cajeput. Mix well together. Rub the parts affected.

RHEUMATIC OIL, NO. II.

Equal proportions of sweet-oil, camphor-water, and hartshorn. Mix well, and rub the parts affected.

REMEDY FOR RHEUMATISM, NO. I.

Take a plant known as wild arsenic, or wild ratsbane; wash the dirt off, and put it, roots and all, into common whiskey, in such quantity that, after steeping twenty-four hours, the liquor will assume a blackish appearance. Rub this on the part diseased, as hard as the pain will allow, for about fifteen minutes; and also have flannel cloths dipped into it, and spread on the parts affected; repeat three times a day. If the pain is much increased while the flannel is on, remove it in ten or fifteen minutes.

REMEDY FOR RHEUMATISM, NO. II.

Take half a pound of sarsaparilla, three ounces of mezereon; three of lignum-vitæ chips, three of lightwood, or pitch-pine knots, and four of sassafras-root. Chop all these woods fine; put them in three gallons of water, and boil to one gallon. When cool, bottle it, adding to each one gill of good spirits, to prevent spoiling. Take one gill of the decoction night and morning, with a teaspoonful of the volatile tincture of guaiacum.

INFALLIBLE CURE FOR DYSENTERY, NO. I.

We can confidently recommend the following recipe in the treatment of dysentery, and other forms of bowel disease: —

Castor-oil, two ounces; bi-carb. soda, one ounce; spirits turpentine, half-ounce; powdered gum-arabic, one ounce; loaf-sugar, one ounce; compound spirits lavender, half-ounce; camphor-water, sufficient to make eight ounces of the mixture.

Dose for an adult—Begin with a teaspoonful every two hours, and increase to a tablespoonful, as the stomach will bear it.

Since dysentery has become one of the most dreaded scourges of the South, and since many of the regular forms of practice have proved unsuccessful in its treatment, we take much pleasure in presenting this prescription to the public. In connection with the above, we advise the use of an occasional opiate, either by mouth or injection, to procure rest and relief from pain. In conclusion, we advise a regular application of hot mustard poultices over the seat of the disease.

CURE FOR DYSENTERY, NO. II.—VERY RELIABLE.

Six ounces of red oak bark, six large pods of red pepper, two ounces of cloves, six ounces of loaf-sugar, two pints of pure spirits, brandy or whiskey. Boil the red oak in a half-gallon of water, until it is reduced to half the quantity. Strain it, and add the pepper, cloves and sugar. Boil together five minutes, and while hot add the spirits. Dose: one tablespoonful for an adult.

DYSENTERY OR FLUX.

Take one pound of gum-arabic, one ounce gum tragacanth. dissolved in two quarts of soft water, and strained. Then take one pound of cloves, half a pound of cinnamon, half a pound of allspice, boil in two quarts of soft water, and strain. Add it to the gums, boil all together over a slow fire, and stir into it two pounds of loaf-sugar. Strain the whole again when you take it off; and when it is cool, add to it a half-pint sweet tincture of rhubarb, and a pint and a half of best brandy. Cork it tight in bottles, as the gums will sour if exposed. If corked properly, it will keep for years.

This is very useful in bowel diseases among children.

FOR CHOLERA MORBUS.

Take spirits of camphor, two tablespoonsful; laudanum, two tablespoonsful; spirits of turpentine, two tablespoonsful; essence of peppermint, one tablespoonful. Mix, and give a teaspoonful every ten or fifteen minutes, until the patient is relieved.

This is an excellent remedy.

FOR CHOLERA.

For premonitory symptoms of cholera, diarrhœa, dysentery, cramp colic, and cholera morbus, the following recipe may be relied on: —

One pint of good brandy, one ounce of laudanum, one ounce of gum camphor, half ounce of Cayenne pepper. Mix well together, and for dose take one teaspoonful.

DIARRHŒA.

Rhubarb, six ounces; catechu, three ounces; ginger, four ounces; cloves, two ounces; spirits of cinnamon, one-fourth of a pint; laudanum, four ounces; spirits of camphor, two ounces; simple syrup, two pints; diluted alcohol, one gallon. Mix, and let it stand fourteen days; then bottle it. Dose: a tablespoonful; repeat according to circumstances.

CHRONIC DIARRHŒA.

To as much blackberry-root as you can grasp in your hand, put two gallons of water, and boil down to half a gallon. Add a tablespoonful of beaten cloves, cinnamon, and enough loaf-sugar to make it sweet. Boil all together, strain, and when cool, add a fourth as much good brandy as you have of the liquor. Take a tablespoonful three times a day, and oftener, if necessary.

FOR BOWEL COMPLAINT.

Take half an ounce of rhubarb, half an ounce of calcined magnesia, and two tablespoonsful of loaf-sugar. Rub these in a mortar, and put them in a bottle. Add one teaspoonful of laudanum; two of essence of mint; two of hartshorn; one tablespoonful of red lavender; two gills of old brandy, and four gills of water. Shake it well before using. Give a dessert spoonful, night and morning, or oftener, if necessary.

RED MIXTURE FOR SUMMER COMPLAINT.

Mix with two ounces of water, two drops of the oil of spearmint, sixteen grains of pulverized rhubarb, thirty of soda, fifty of prepared chalk, and cork tightly. A teaspoonful for a child, tablespoonful for a grown person.

COLIC.

An attack of colic is often instantly relieved, by the following dose:—

Castor-oil, two tablespoonsful; laudanum, one teaspoonful; spirits of turpentine, one tablespoonful. Take the above for one dose, and repeat, if necessary.

CURE FOR COLIC.

One ounce of cloves, two ounces of cinnamon, two ounces of ginger-root pared, two ounces of allspice, three drachms oil of lavender, one and a half pints of alcohol; pulverize and mix together. Set it in the sun for ten days, shake often, then strain, and it will be fit for use. Dose: a teaspoonful on sugar, according to circumstances, till relief is obtained.

FOR CLEANSING AND PURIFYING THE BLOOD.

Take one pound of sarsaparilla, a half-pound of guaiacum shavings, one ounce of sassafras, half-pound of elder-flowers, half-pound of alder-buds, half-pound of burdock-root; put all these together, and add two quarts of boiling water to one-third of it. Take a wine-glassful three times a day, and a dose of pills once or twice a week.

FOR RING-WORM, SHINGLES, AND SOME OTHER DISEASES OF THE SKIN.

Tincture of Spanish flies, one ounce and a half; kreosote, one drachm; acetic acid, a half-ounce; oil of bergamot, ten drops; mix together. When used, the vial should be well shaken. Apply by moistening the end of the finger, or a small rag, and rub the parts affected three times a day. This daily application should be continued until small blisters, or pimples, appear, when it should be discontinued. The disease is generally cured when the blisters dry up: should the cure not be effected, apply the medicine the second time, as at first.

REMEDY FOR ITCH, NO. I.

Brown soap, one ounce; common salt, half an ounce; sulphur, half an ounce; alcohol, a teaspoonful; vinegar, a tablespoonful; chloride of lime, a half drachm. Rub well together; one-fourth to be used, night and morning, as a friction. It is effectual, cheap, and inoffensive.

REMEDY FOR ITCH, NO. II.

Take black pepper, ginger, and brimstone, each of equal parts; a little West India rum, and a little lard: all well mixed, as a salve. Rub a little on your hands, hold them to the fire, and smell for a few minutes; repeat it several times a day.

RING-WORMS.

Rub mercurial ointment on, at night, and repeat it, as often as is necessary.

CURE FOR TETTER, OR RING-WORM.

After I had the tetter-worm for nearly twenty years on my hand, a friend advised me to take some blood-root, (called also red-root, Indian paint, &c.,) slice it in vinegar, and afterward wash the place affected, with the liquid. I suppose the vinegar extracted the strength out of the root, for in a few days the dry scurf was removed, and my diseased hand appeared as whole as the other. I could scarcely believe that a perfect cure was so speedily accomplished by this simple remedy; but as nearly two years have passed without the least appearance of its return, I need no longer doubt the fact, and for the benefit of others I wish the value of the red-root more generally known.

The red-root grows about a foot high in rich woodland, and flowers in April. The leaf is roundish and deeply indented, somewhat like the white-oak leaves, stems naked, supporting single flowers, blossoms white. When the fresh root, which is about the size of the little finger, and blood-red, is broken, a juice issues in large drops resembling blood.

SALT RHEUM.

Take one quart of tar; add two gallons of water; let it stand two or three days, stirring it occasionally; then soak, or pour off the water, and put into bottles. Take half a teacupful three times a day, before eating. The following ointment should be made and used externally, while drinking tar-water: — Take the yolk of an egg; the same size, of fresh butter; half the size, of tar; one teaspoonful pulverized cream of tartar. Mix them together with the point of a knife, until it becomes a perfect salve. Anoint the parts affected three times a day with this ointment, and the cure is effected in two weeks.

PRICKLY HEAT.

Mix a good proportion of wheat bran with tepid water, and bathe with it three times a day, or if necessary, oftener.

A CURE FOR THRUSH.

The root called Hog's Tush may be mashed fine, and steeped in a little water for two or three hours; then the mouth may be washed with the liquor, sweetened with sugar, two or three times in the course of a day. This is a never-failing remedy, and generally two or three applications are sufficient.

RUNROUND.

When the first symptoms of swelling and inflammation appear, place the finger firm, and with a sharp-pointed knife, scratch the nail crosswise, and then lengthwise, leaving the whole surface rough and white. If neglected till it begins to suppurate, open it with a needle, and *then* scratch the nail.

CURE FOR A WEN.

Make a very strong brine, and dip in it a piece of flannel two or three times doubled, and apply it to the wen, keeping it constantly wet, night and day, until a suppuration takes place.

A SALVE AND WASH FOR ULCERS.

Salve. — One ounce of rosin.
Two ounces of bees-wax.
Four ounces of hog's lard.

To be simmered together well mixed.

Wash. — One teaspoonful fine salt.
One teaspoonful pulverized alum.

Put into one pint of red shank tea, made pretty strong. The ulcer is to be well cleaned with this wash, wiped dry, and the place well filled up with fine lint; then apply a plaster of the salve. A fresh plaster should be applied every morning.

TO CURE A CANCER BY EXTRACTING IT.

Take oxyde of arsenic, and flour of sulphur, each one drachm; spermaceti ointment, one ounce; add all together, and make an ointment, and apply some of it, spread on lint, to the ulcer; let it remain twenty-four hours; then press the ulcer with a soft poultice, or simple salve. If necessary, repeat it.

CURE FOR A CANCER.

Take the narrow-leafed dock-root, and boil it in water till it be quite soft; then bathe the part affected in the decoction, as hot as can be borne, three or four times a day; the root must then be mashed and applied as a poultice.

AN EFFECTUAL CURE FOR A FELON.

Bathe the part affected in ashes and water; take the yolk of an egg, six drops of spirits of turpentine a few beet-leaves cut fine, a small quantity of hard soap, one teaspoonful of snuff, or fine tobacco; then add one tablespoonful of burned salt, and one of Indian-meal; it never fails to effect a cure, if applied in season.

ANOTHER.

Take of rock, or any other table-salt, one ounce; hard soap, one ounce; spirits of turpentine, half an ounce; roast the salt, rolled in a cabbage-leaf or wet paper, for twenty or thirty minutes, then pulverize it; mix with the soap, previously shaved down, and add the spirits of turpentine, which will make a soft salve or poultice. This must be applied to the affected part, and renewed as often as it becomes dry. If applied before it suppurates, it will prevent the formation of matter by three or four hours' application; if not applied until suppuration begins, it will stop its progress; but the matter must be let out, when the ulcer will be healed by the same means as in any other case of the like kind.

CURE FOR THE POLYPUS IN THE NOSE.

Take one half-ounce of blood-root finely pulverized, and sift it, and one drachm of calomel; mix them together for a sternutatory. A small pinch of this powder is to be snuffed up the nostril three times a day, and a syringe of the following wash is to be thrown up the nostrils twice a day:—Dissolve half an ounce of powdered alum in a gill of brandy; shake the vial until it is dissolved.

ANOTHER.

Take of blood-root and bayberry-root bark, equal parts mixed, made fine, and used as a snuff several times a day.

CURE FOR THE DROPSY, NO. I.

Take cinders from a blacksmith's shop, and beat them fine, sift them, and take out the coarse particles; mix the fine cinders with a pint of honey, until it is stiff enough to lie on the point of a case-knife, not hard like pills. Give the patient as much as will lie on the point of a case-knife, three times a day, morning, noon, and night. This mixture is very purgative, and will cause the patient to discharge great quantities of water, both purgatively and by urine. The potion may be given according to the operation: if the quantity appears to be too severe, give less; if it does not operate enough, give more, and continue it until the swelling is gone.

The patient may eat any diet but milk, of which he should not taste a drop; neither use any other medicine while taking the above.

CURE FOR THE DROPSY, NO. II.

Sulphate of potash, two ounces; cream of tartar, two ounces; powdered squills, one drachm; tartar emetic, one grain. Mix the whole. Dose: a tablespoonful two or three times a day, until it operates on the bowels; then a spoonful; and if it does not operate, add a tablespoonful of jalap to the whole mixture.

CURE FOR JAUNDICE, NO. I.

Rhubarb root, gum aloes, orange-peel, canella bark, gentian root, columbo root, coriander seed, of each two drachms. Bruise, and add a quart of good spirits. To prevent chills, add three or four drachms of Peruvian bark. Dose: a tablespoonful three or four times a day.

CURE FOR JAUNDICE, NO. II.

Take of the bark of the wild-cherry tree, and the bark of sassafras root, which steep in good rum, and take a glass in the morning.

CURE FOR WORMS IN CHILDREN.

The following preparation, after long and satisfactory experience, is confidently recommended as a certain cure for worms: — Take the fat of old bacon, sliced, and fried in a pan until the essence is all out of it; take out the rind first, then put in as much wormseed (commonly called Jerusalem oak) as is necessary, as much sugar or molasses as will make it palatable, and give it three mornings in succession. The children will eat it freely; some you will have to restrain from eating too much. Incredible as it may appear, I have known as many as one hundred and twenty or thirty large worms come from a child three or four years old. I usually give the medicine in the spring and fall.

ANOTHER FOR WORMS.

Butternut syrup, one tablespoonful; composition, two tablespoonsful; castor-oil, one tablespoonful. Give in small doses until relief is obtained.

CURE FOR THE GRAVEL, NO. I.

Drink strong coffee, without sugar or milk. This dissolves the gravel, and allows it to pass off, with very little pain.

CURE FOR THE GRAVEL, NO. II.

Make a strong tea of blackberry brier-root; add some Virginia snake-root; while this is steeping, give the patient freely of cayenne or composition powders; then drink freely of the tea, and in fifteen minutes after drinking this tea, give two teaspoonsful of the pulverized butterfly or pleurisy root, in a teacupful of hot water, sweetened; repeat both every half-hour alternately for ten or twelve hours; then use a tea of parsley three or four days.

For strengthening and invigorating the nerves, one ounce juniper-berries, two ounces orris-root, one ounce bitter bugle, and three ounces camomile flowers; break them up fine; steep one tablespoonful in half a pint of boiling water, and drink it through the day. Take a gentle purgative once or twice a week, if the bowels are at all constipated.

A SHRUNKEN SINEW, OR STIFF JOINT.

Mix half an ounce each, of green melilot, yellow basilicon, oil of amber, and a piece of blue vitriol as large as a thimble; simmer well together over a slow fire, in two ounces of lard, to the consistency of salve; apply it to the shrunken part and the joint next above, at least three times a day, rubbing it well.

HEADACHE DROPS.

For the cure of nervous, sun, and sick head-ache, take two quarts of alcohol, three ounces Castile soap, one ounce camphor, and two ounces ammonia. Bathe the forehead and temples.

CURE FOR THE SCARLET FEVER.

As soon as the nature of the disease is ascertained, commence rubbing the patient with a piece of fat bacon, until the surface of the whole body is saturated with the grease. Take a piece of bacon with the rind on, as it is thus more convenient to handle, and rub thoroughly twice a-day. It is well to slit the soft side of the bacon, as the fat will thus be enabled to run more freely.

Greasing the throat and breast alone, in this manner, has proved beneficial.

Avoid the use of calomel, and all other violent remedies.

PREVENTIVE OF SCARLET FEVER.

Dissolve three grains of the extract of belladonna in one ounce of cinnamon-water (triturated together in a mortar), and of this solution give three drops in a little sugar and water, to a child one year old, once a day, increasing the dose one drop for every additional year. In this minute dose it can do no possible injury; whilst the mass of evidence in favor of its complete prophylactic power, is conclusive. This has been used with great success.

CURE FOR CONSUMPTION, NO. I.

A temperate mode of living (avoiding spirituous liquors wholly), wearing flannel next to the skin, and taking every morning half a pint of new milk, mixed with the expressed juice of green hoarhound, will not only relieve the complaints, but the patient shall procure to himself a length of days beyond what the mildest fever could give room to hope for.

Four weeks' use of the hoarhound and milk have relieved the pains of the breast, and enabled the patient to breathe deep, long, and free; strengthened and harmonized the voice; and restored him to a better state of health than he had enjoyed for many years.

CURE FOR CONSUMPTION, NO. II.

Take three quarts of good spring-water, a quart of wheat bran, and half a pint of honey; simmer them gently for two or three hours, in a stone pot, over a slow fire. Let the compound cool sufficiently to admit yeast through it; then put in half a pint of good yeast, and let it stand thirty-six hours. Take half a wine-glass three times a day, a few minutes before eating. If this appears too much, take a less quantity. To the use of this, a consumptive confidently ascribes his rescue from an early grave, to which he was fast hastening, by a consumption brought on by the measles.

CHILLS AND FEVER.

Gum myrrh, twenty-four grains; gum assafœtida, twenty-four grains; blue mass, twenty-four grains; quinine, forty-eight grains; oil of black pepper, sufficient to mix. Divide into twenty-four pills. Dose, one pill three or four times a day.

NEURALGIA.

Quinine, five grains; precipitated carbonate of iron, four grains; morphine, half a grain; mix with syrup, and take at one dose. Should it fail to relieve in an hour, repeat it.

FOR PALPITATION OF THE HEART.

Take ten drops traumatic balsam, two or three times a day, on sugar.

CURE FOR DEAFNESS, NO. I.

It is said that by melting sulphuric ether and ammonia, and allowing it to stand fourteen days, a solution is formed, which, if properly applied to the internal ear, will remove, in almost every case, this hitherto considered incurable affection.

CURE FOR DEAFNESS, NO. II.

Equal parts of the juice of houseleek, brandy, and sweet-oil, in a vial, to be hung up exposed to the sun for a month or more. This dropped in the ear at night, and on wool to be kept in the ear, is a sure remedy for deafness.

CURE FOR DEAFNESS, NO. III.

Syringe the ears well with some warm milk and oil, then take a quarter of an ounce of liquid opodeldoc, and as much oil of almonds; mix them well, and drop a few drops into each ear, stopping them with a little cotton or wool: repeat this every night when going to bed.

CURE FOR THE GOUT.

The best cure for the gout is to apply a leek poultice to the part affected; numerous instances of its efficacy in this painful disorder have recently occurred.

CORDIAL FOR WEAK STOMACHS.

An excellent article to strengthen and restore the tone of the stomach. It prevents faintness, or a sinking feeling at the stomach; and for persons subject to low and depressed spirits, it affords great relief. It is made thus:—

Dissolve, of gum-arabic, two ounces, in one pint of rain-water, and add one and a half wine-glasses of best brandy. Take a tablespoonful three or four times a day.

STRENGTHENING PLASTER.

Take of resin, beeswax, white turpentine, one pound each; one tablespoonful of black pepper, pulverized; one pint of French brandy. Put the whole into a new earthen crock; melt and simmer till the brandy is all evaporated.

ANOTHER may be made by melting turpentine with a sufficient quantity of resin to give it a proper consistence.

CURE FOR SWELLED OR INFLAMED BREASTS, NO. I.

Take soft-soap, and make strong suds, and with a flannel cloth, saturated with the suds, wash and rub the breast downward with some degree of violence, once an hour; after which each time bathe the breast with polecat oil, or some soft grease and camphor. Keep the breast close covered with flannel.

CURE FOR SWELLED OR INFLAMED BREASTS, NO. II.

Take hard soap and common salt, each two ounces; new milk, half a pint; shave the soap fine; put all into a vessel, and simmer slowly over a fire. Take care not to burn. When hot, stir in a spoonful of corn meal. Spread all on one cloth, and cover the whole breast. The surface of the poultice should be covered with soft grease, and the plaster should be applied as hot as can be borne. A new poultice to be applied every three hours, till relief is given.

EYE-WATER, FOR CURE OF SORE EYES.

Take white vitriol, a lump about the size of a pea; and a lump twice that size of loaf-sugar; three cloves, pulverized, and well mixed; a hen's egg, roasted or boiled very hard; peel off the shell, cut through the middle, and take out the yolk; put the aforesaid powder into the hollow where the yolk was; place the two halves of the egg together again, wrap it in a strong cloth, and wring it hard; do not have too much cloth around the egg; wring quickly; drop one drop of the juice in the eye, or dip the finger in the liquid, and touch the corner of the eye.

ANOTHER—FOR CHRONIC SORE EYES.

One ounce lobelia seed, one ounce Cayenne pepper seed, one ounce gum myrrh, one ounce lady's slipper, half an ounce camphor, and of alcohol one pint; pulverize and mix them together, set it in the sun ten days, shake it often, and strain it in a bottle for use.

FOR INFLAMED OR WEAK EYES.

Half-fill a pint bottle with common table salt. Fill it up with good French brandy. Shake it, let it settle, and bathe the outside of the eye with a soft linen cloth, on going to bed, and occasionally through the day. It is a good application for pains and bruises generally.

EAR ACHE.

Take a large onion, bore a hole two-thirds through, large enough to contain a tablespoonful of sweet-oil; roast and press out the juice, add a little laudanum, wet a piece of cotton with the liquid, and put it in the ear.

POULTICES.

1. A good poultice may be made of crumbs of bread boiled with milk, sweet-oil, or spring-water.

2. Brown sugar and soap make a good poultice, or salve, for a boil.

3. Four ounces of white lily roots, a pound of figs, and four ounces of meal or bean flour, boiled together, with as much water as will cover them, make an excellent poultice for swellings and suppurating sores.

4. For cancers, or running sores, a grated carrot, boiled quite soft, makes a good poultice.

5. Salad leaves, well boiled, make a poultice that relieves pain.

6. Flaxseed, or camomile flowers, boiled with the tops of worm-wood, make an excellent poultice for inflammations.

7. A stimulating poultice is made by using vinegar instead of water, and the addition of garlic, mustard, horse-radish, &c., to crumbs of bread, or to flour.

LIQUID COMPOUNDS, FOR THE CURE AND PREVENTION OF BALDNESS.

1. Oil of mace, a half-ounce; olive-oil, two drachms; water of ammoniac, a half-drachm; spirits of rosemary, one ounce; rose-water, two and a half ounces. Mix.

2. Eau de Cologne, two ounces; tincture of cantharides, two drachms; oil of rosemary, and oil of lavender, of each ten drops.

3. Equal parts of rectified spirits, castor-oil, and eau de Cologne.

4. Equal parts of honey-water, and tincture of cantharides.

5. Tincture of cantharides, three drachms; acetate of copper, three grains; oil of almonds, and castor-oil, of each a fluid ounce; with an essential oil to scent it. A small quantity to be applied to the roots of the hair every morning.

6. Vinegar of cantharides, half an ounce; of eau de Cologne, one ounce; rose-water, one ounce. Mix.

7. Castor-oil, lavender-water, and tincture of cantharides, in equal quantities.

8. Bay leaves, two ounces; cloves, one-fourth of an ounce; spirits of lavender, four ounces; spirits of thyme, four ounces; and add a half-ounce of ether. To be rubbed on every morning.

AMERICAN SHAMPOO LIQUID.

Rum, three quarts; spirits of wine, one pint; tincture of cantharides, half an ounce; carbonate of ammonia, half-ounce; salt of tartar, one ounce.

The foregoing ointments and liquids require to be used for some weeks, in order to produce a decided effect, either in curing or preventing baldness.

Those which contain cantharides in any form are the most active, and must be used with caution. They should be applied once or twice a day, according to the effect produced; but if the scalp becomes sore, their use must be intermitted for a time, or longer intervals allowed, as the case may require. When employed to prevent the hair falling off, or becoming grey, they need not be applied so frequently as for baldness.

WASHES FOR THE HAIR.

1. Southern-wood, two ounces; box-leaves, six ounces; water, four pints. Boil gently in a saucepan for a quarter of an hour; strain, and to each pint of the liquid add two ounces of rosemary, and a half drachm of salt of tartar, or one drachm of Naples soap.

2. Boil one pound of rosemary in two quarts of water, and add to the filtered liquor one ounce of spirits of lavender, and one-fourth of an ounce of Naples soap, or salt of tartar.

3. Incinerate two ounces each, of rosemary, maidenhair, southern-wood, myrtle berries, and hazel bark. Make a strong solution of the ashes, with which wash the hair at the roots every day. Keep the hair short.

4. *Wash for Removing Scurf, and Promoting the Curling of the Hair.*—Beat up the yolk of an egg with a pint of clear rain-water. Apply it warm, and afterwards wash the head with warm water.

GERMAN POMADE FOR STRENGTHENING THE HAIR.

Take eight ounces of purified marrow, melt it in a glass or stone jar, and add one and a half ounces of fresh bay leaves, one ounce of orange leaves, one ounce of bitter almonds, a half-ounce of nutmegs, a half-ounce of cloves, and one drachm of vanilla, all bruised. Cover the vessel, and let the whole digest for twenty-four hours, with a gentle heat. Strain, while warm, through linen, and stir it as it cools.

POMADES FOR BEAUTIFYING THE HAIR.

1. *Common Pomatum.*—Mutton suet, one pound; prepared lard, three pounds. Melt together, pour it it into an earthen basin, and beat it assiduously with a wooden spatula. When cool, add two ounces of bergamot, or of lemon, and continue the stirring until nearly cold.

2. *Rose Pomatum.*—Prepared lard, sixteen ounces; prepared suet, two ounces. Melt with a gentle heat, and add two ounces of rose-water, and six drops of attar of roses. Beat them well together, and put it into pots before it gets too cold.

For making jessamine, violet and orange pomades, put the same quantity of water, and one drachm of the essence.

3. *Marrow Pomatum.*—Beef marrow and beef suet, mixed together, and boiled gently for a short time.

4. Oil of sweet almonds, a pint; spermaceti, one and a half ounces; purified lard, two ounces. Melt with a gentle heat. When nearly cold, add any agreeable scent, and pour it into pots, or wide-mouthed bottles.

VETERINARY RECEIPTS.

LENGTH OF ANIMAL LIFE.

A HARE will live ten years; a cat, ten; a goat, eight; an ox, twenty; a hog, twenty-five; a pigeon, eight; a turtle-dove, twenty-five; a raven, one hundred; an eagle, one hundred; and a goose, one hundred and fifty.

GESTATION.

The period of gestation, or the length of time which different animals go with young, should be known by every farmer, that the season of copulation with his different kinds of stock may be so regulated as to have them bring forth their young under the most favorable circumstances.

Mares go a few days over eleven months with foal. Cows go about forty weeks, or ten lunar months. Ewes bring forth at the end of five months. Goats, at four and a half months. Sows, at four months.

The term of incubation, or time which different fowls sit upon their eggs before hatching, is as follows: —

Swans sit six weeks; turkeys sit thirty days; geese, from twenty-seven to thirty days; ducks, from twenty-seven to thirty days; hens, twenty-one days; pigeons, or doves, fifteen days.

28

TO JUDGE THE AGE OF A HORSE BY HIS TEETH.

At two years old, the horse sheds the two middle teeth of the under jaw. At three years old, he sheds two other teeth, one on each side of those he shed the year before. At four years old, he sheds the two remaining, or corner teeth. At five years old, the two middle teeth are full, no longer hollow as all the others are, and the teeth have penetrated the gums. At six years old, the four middle teeth are full, the corner teeth only remaining hollow; the tusks are sharp, with the sides fluted. At seven years old, the corner teeth are full, the tusks longer and thicker, and the horse is said to be aged.

It is not meant that, exactly at the period mentioned, these changes take place in the horse: much depends upon his constitution, and whether he be a late or early foal: also upon the manner in which he has been reared, as to food, shelter, &c. The corner tooth, too, might remain a little hollow after the age of seven, but the appearance is still very unlike the mere shells which they are at the age of six.

AGE OF SHEEP

May be known by examining the front teeth. They are eight in number, and appear, during the first year, of a small size. In the second year, the two middle ones fall out, and their place is supplied by two new teeth, which are easily distinguished by their being of a larger size. In the third year, the two other small teeth, one from each side, drop out, and are replaced by two larger ones; so that there are four large teeth in the middle, and two pointed ones on each side. In the fourth year, the large teeth are six in number, and only two small ones remain, one at each end of the range. In the fifth year, the remaining small teeth are lost, and the whole front teeth are larger. In the sixth year, the whole begin to be worn; and in the seventh, sometimes sooner, some fall out or are broken.

TO PREVENT HORSES BEING TEASED BY FLIES.

Take two or three small handsful of walnut leaves, upon which pour two or three quarts of cold water; let it infuse one night; pour the whole, next morning, into a kettle, and let it boil for a quarter of an hour. When cold, it will be fit for use. No more is required than to moisten a sponge, and before the horse goes out of the stable, let those parts which are most irritable be smeared over with the liquor, viz: between and upon the ears, the neck, flank, &c. Not only the lady or gentleman, who rides out for pleasure, will derive benefit from the walnut leaves thus prepared, but the coachman, the wagoner, and all who use horses during the hot months.

SORE TONGUE IN HORSES—A PRETTY CERTAIN CURE.

Dissolve two ounces of copperas, and two of alum, in a pint of strong vinegar; swab the mouth and tongue with the solution until the disease is removed. Then dissolve honey and alum in vinegar, and use it in the same way to heal the tongue.

ANOTHER, FOR SORE TONGUE IN HORSES.

Make a strong decoction of red-oak bark, and when cold, dissolve a small quantity of alum and copperas in it. Then wash the tongue, or pour the liquid in the mouth with a bottle; hold it a while, and let the horse throw it out.

LINIMENT FOR THE GALLED BACKS OF HORSES.

Keating, in his expedition to the source of St. Peter's River, says:—For the information of other travellers, we may mention, that, after having tried many applications to the backs of horses, when galled, we have found none that succeeded so well as white-lead moistened with milk. When milk was not to be procured, oil was substituted. Whenever the application was made in the early stage of the wound, we have found it to be very effectual, and it is likewise a convenient one, as two ounces of white-lead sufficed for the whole of our party for more than a month.

SADDLE GALLS.

Saddle galls are generally occasioned by an unequal pressure of the saddle, or by a saddle being badly fitted to a horse's back, and if neglected they grow into very ugly and troublesome sores. When these inflamed tumors are first discovered, cold water alone is frequently sufficient to disperse and drive them away; but when that will not have the desired effect, the back may be washed twice a day in a mixture of sharp vinegar, one gill; spirits of any kind, one gill; sweet-oil, or fresh butter, one tablespoonful; to be well mixed before used.

SWELLINGS ON HORSES OR CATTLE.

To scatter swellings on horses or cattle, take two quarts of proof whiskey, or other proof spirits; warm it over coals, but not to blaze; dissolve it in a pint of soft-soap; when cool put it in a bottle, and add one ounce of camphor. When dissolved, it will form the liquid opodeldoc, and is then ready for application, making a cheap and useful remedy. When the swelling is on the leg, or any part that will receive a bandage, such bandage should be applied, and wet with the opodeldoc.

KING'S OIL FOR CURING WOUNDS ON HORSES AND CATTLE.

One ounce of green copperas, two ounces of white vitriol, two ounces of common salt, two ounces of linseed oil, and eight ounces of molasses; pulverize the copperas, and boil all over a slow fire fifteen minutes in a pint of wine. When almost cold, add one ounce oil of vitriol, and four ounces spirits of turpentine. Apply to the wound with a quill or feather. This will immediately set the wound to running, and perform a certain cure.

TO CURE SWINNEY.

Get a bottle of fresh turpentine; curry and brush the part affected; then rub with the turpentine from the top of the shoulder-blade downwards, about nine inches, and if the horse is much affected by it, in eight or ten hours grease the parts with lard, and repeat the turpentine in three days again. In stubborn cases, stick an awl in the sunken part to the bone, in two or three places, and apply the turpentine, and then, with a warm iron, plat the parts, or, as it is termed, "bake in the turpentine."

ANOTHER REMEDY

Is to make a small incision in the sunken or perished part of the shoulder, near the uppermost point; then, with the barrel of a goose-quill, blow up the part affected, till a large puff is made round about; in the mean time, with the sides of the hands striking or pressing the air under the skin in every direction. Then close the hole effectually with a pin, and hair tied around the same. With proper rest to the horse, he may be regarded as cured. Repeat the blowing of the air or wind on successive days; it is to prevent the pressure of the skin on the part affected. Let a second person place the end of his finger on the end of the quill, while securing the air.

ANOTHER REMEDY.

Bathing the part affected with saltpetre dissolved in water, has been known to effect a complete cure.

CRACKS IN THE HEELS, OR WOUNDS IN HORSES.

Sugar of lead, two drachms; white vitriol, one drachm; and a strong infusion of red-oak bark, or elm, all well mixed together. Wash or bathe the parts affected with the above preparation.

LOST APPETITE IN A HORSE.

Horses lose their appetites from various causes, viz: excessive fatigue, want of a change in food, dirty fodder, moldy corn, or a dirty manger, &c.;—but most frequently by the approach of some disease. So soon as you discover a horse has lost his appetite, observe the following treatment, viz:—Take from the neck vein half a gallon of blood; then take of assafœtida, a quarter of an ounce; salt, one tablespoonful; sassafras tea, one quart. Mix, and give him a drench. On the second day, take of glauber salts, one pound; warm water, one quart. After dissolving the salts, give it as a drench, and in two or three days the appetite will be restored, unless the animal is laboring under some disease which may be ascertained by the symptoms.

ANOTHER REMEDY.

Take half a pound of saltpeter, half a pound of alum, and half a pound of alum salt; pulverize and mix them well together, and every eight or ten days give the horse a tablespoonful in his food. His coat, flesh, and spirits will soon reward his master for his care.

MASH FOR HORSES.

A mash is generally given to a horse for the purpose of cooling the system, opening the bowels, and for disguising different kinds of medicine, which may be necessary to be administered, and which, if given in any other way, would be attended with difficulty, and would be unproductive of effects so salutary.

Mash No. 1. Take of bran, one gallon; sassafras tea (scalding hot), one quart; powdered brimstone, one tablespoonful; saltpeter, one teaspoonful.

No. 2. Take oats, one gallon; flour of sulphur, one tablespoonful; saltpeter, one teaspoonful; boiling water, one quart.

No. 3. Take of bran, one gallon; glauber salts, four ounces; sulphur, one tablespoonful; sassafras tea (scalding hot), one quart. Let them be well mixed, and given milk-warm, not permitting the horse to drink cold water for six hours afterward.

BLISTERS.

Previous to the application of a blister to any part of a horse, the hair should either be shaved or cut off as close as possible; the blistering ointment should be regularly spread with a warm knife on a stout piece of osnaburg; and during the operation of the blister, the horse should be tied short to prevent his biting the part, or doing other injury.

Blister No. 1. Take of Spanish flies, half an ounce; oil of turpentine, one ounce; hog's lard, four ounces; mix them well, and the blister is ready for use.

No. 2. Take of tar, four ounces; vitriol acid, two drachms; oil of origanum, half an ounce; hog's lard, two ounces; Spanish flies, two ounces. This blister is excellent for the spavin.

CLYSTER.

As clysters very often are the means of saving horses' lives, I shall here recommend the best and simplest method of administering them. Take a large bladder, cut off the neck, and soften it in warm water. Take a pewter pipe, common reed, or any other smooth tube, nine or ten inches long, and not more than an inch in diameter; the clyster must then be poured through a funnel into the bag, and securely tied around one end of the tube; the other must be made perfectly smooth and rounded, well oiled, and introduced into the anus several inches; the liquor in the bladder must be forced through the tube by pressure with the hand. When a clyster is given, a horse should be placed with his head down hill, and if he refuses to stand, a twitch should be put upon his nose.

Clysters are of three kinds — opening, anodyne, and nourishing. For the first purpose take a gallon of warm water, with from half a pound to a pound of common salt dissolved in it; to which add four or five ounces of linseed oil. For the second take two drachms of solid opium, dissolve them, or rather mix them well with about half a pint of warm water, and add from a quart to three pints of Indian-meal, or wheat flour gruel. For the third purpose, rich broths, wheat flour gruel, and other nourishing fluids, are recommended.

With respect to the first kind of clysters, it may be observed that gruel is commonly preferred to warm water; but, according to my experience, the latter does just as well as the former. As to the second, tincture of opium may be substituted for solid opium, and is by some preferred to it; but the quantity should not exceed two ounces, on account of the spirit in which this opium is dissolved. The third kind of clyster is required only in lock-jaw, or in diseases of the throat which prevent swallowing, and in these its utility seems to be very questionable.

As soon as the clyster has been injected, the tail should be kept close to the fundament for a few minutes, to prevent its being too hastily returned. This is particularly necessary when the anodyne clyster has been employed. The pipe must be oiled, or greased, before it is introduced; and if its passage be obstructed by hard excrement lodged in the rectum, the hand should be gradually introduced in order to remove it.

CURE FOR THE SCOURS IN HORSES.

Put into a junk bottle one pint of good gin, and one ounce of indigo; shake well together, and pour it down the horse's throat.

COLIC IN HORSES, NO. I.

Jamestown seed, from four to ten tablespoonsful, boiled, and poured off, given to a horse, will effect a cure in ten or fifteen minutes. Bleed the horse in the mouth.

COLIC IN HORSES, NO. II.

Make and give him a drench composed of a tablespoonful of strong mustard, dissolved in a pint of water, which may be administered in a black junk bottle, by raising the horse's head a sufficient height. If it be uncertain when the horse was first affected, as in that case there will be danger of inflammation, on discovery of the disorder, bleed a vein immediately. The remedy here described is said to be immediate and infallible.

COLIC IN HORSES, NO. III.

I was lately told by a gentleman of Prince George county, that a teacupful of spirits of turpentine would give instant relief to horses laboring under this disorder. He added that, on one occasion, all the oxen of two of his carts were suddenly swollen by the generation of gas in the stomach, from eating green food. The overseer expected all would die, when our informant ordered a teacupful of spirits of turpentine, diffused in oil, to be given to each. The relief was in every case instantaneous and effectual, almost before he could have thought there was time to swallow. Such facts should always be communicated for wide diffusion and preservation.

COLIC, OR GRIPES.

Symptoms. — The symptoms of the colic commence with great restlessness and uneasiness in the horse's manner of standing; frequently he paws, voids small quantities of excrement, and makes many fruitless attempts to stale; kicks his belly with his hind legs; often looks round to his flanks, groaning, expressive of the pain he feels; lies down, rolls, gets up again, and sometimes for a moment appears to find relief. But the pain soon returns with double violence; his ears are generally cold, and he often sweats about the flank and shoulders; his body swells, and he frequently shows a disposition to lie down in great haste.

A TABLE FOR DISTINGUISHING

Between the Colic, or Gripes, and Inflammation of the Bowels of Horses, by the symptoms that mark the character of each.

SPASMODIC OR FLATULENT COLIC.	INFLAMMATION OF THE BOWELS.
1. Pulse natural, though sometimes a little lower. (1.)	1. Pulse very quick and small. (2.)
2. The horse lies down and rolls upon his back.	2. He lies down and suddenly rises up again, seldom rolling upon his back.
3. The legs and ears are generally warm.	3. Legs and ears generally cold.
4. Attacks suddenly, is never preceded, and seldom accompanied, by any symptoms of fever.	4. In general, inflammation comes on gradually, is commonly preceded, and always accompanied by symptoms of fever.
5. There are frequently short intermissions.	5. No intermission can be observed.

(1.) Pulse natural.—When in health, the pulsations or strokes are from thirty-six to forty in a minute; those of large heavy horses being slower than those of smaller; and those of old ones slower than those of young animals. When either are just off a quick pace, the strokes increase in number; as they do if he be alarmed or animated by the familiar cry of the hounds.

(2.) Pulse very quick and small.—Fever of the simple or common kind usually increases the pulsations to double the healthy number; as the fever increases in violence, and particularly in cases of inflammation of the bowels, the pulse beats still higher, and reaches to a hundred or more in a minute. To ascertain either state, the attendant should apply the points of his fingers gently to the artery which lies nearest the surface. Some prefer consulting the temporal artery, which is situated about an inch and a half backward from the corner of the eye. Others again, and they are the greatest number, think it best to feel it underneath the edge of the jaw-bone, where the facial artery passes on under the skin only to the side of the face. In either case, too great pressure would stop the pulsation altogether; though such a trial of the artery against the jaw-bone, will prove whether it be in such a rigid state of excitement as attends high fever; or elastic and springy, slipping readily from under the finger, as it does when health prevails, and the strokes follow each other regularly. The presence of high fever is farther indicated by a kind of twang, or vibration, given by the pulse against the finger-points, resembling such as would be felt were we to take hold of a distended whip-cord or wire between the fingers and cause it to vibrate like a fiddle-string, sharply; whereas, in health, a swell is felt in the vibration as if the string were made of soft materials, and not so tightly drawn. Languid or slow pulse, scarcely perceptible in some of the beats or strokes, indicates lowness of spirits, debility, or exhaustion: if languor be felt at intervals only, a few strokes being very quick, and then again a few very slow, this indicates low fever, in which bleeding would do no harm, &c.

Remedies.—1. Take from the neck vein half a gallon of blood; then take of laudanum one ounce, and of mint tea one quart, milk warm; mix them well in a bottle, and give the contents as a drench; let the horse be well rubbed under the belly, and prepare and give an injection of meal, water, molasses, salt, and hog's lard, milk warm.

2. Take of mint tea one and a half pints; gin, or any spirituous liquor, half a pint; mix them well in a bottle, and give them as a drench, taking care to rub the horse well. Should it not have the desired effect in fifteen minutes, repeat the dose.

3. Take of camphor a quarter of an ounce, oil of turpentine half an ounce, mint tea one pint; mix them in a bottle and give them as a drench; confine the horse in a close stable, cover him with three or four blankets, and under his belly place a large tub of boiling water, which will readily throw him into a profuse sweat, and relieve him from pain.

4. In addition to the above, clysters ought to be administered by injecting the following ingredients, viz: water, half a gallon; salt, one handful; oil of any kind, one pint; molasses, one pint; mix the whole and

inject it; and repeat it every half hour, until the bowels are well opened.

FOUNDER IN HORSES, NO. I.

A founder evidently proceeds from surfeit; a horse ridden until heated and fatigued, and fed too plentifully while warm and hungry, and swallowing his food too greedily, that he may lie down and rest his wearied limbs, while the stable is wet or damp, and the horse in a copious sweat, are the best reasons that can be given for the formation of the disease. Instead of rising up refreshed, the poor animal is stiff and useless. If he had been allowed to cool perfectly, and then fed sparingly, he would have escaped this sore complaint.

The remedy is a lump of alum, the size of a walnut, reduced to powder and dissolved in warm water; the horse must be drenched with this liquid, which in a short time will throw him into a profuse perspiration, and he will be able to pursue his journey the next day, or if not badly foundered, in a few hours.

FOUNDER IN HORSES, NO. II.

So soon as you are convinced that your horse is foundered, take from his neck-vein at least one gallon of blood; give a drench of one quart of strong sassafras tea, one teaspoonful of saltpeter, and a quarter of an ounce of assafœtida, and do not permit him to eat or drink for five or six hours; at the expiration of which time, should he not be evidently better, repeat the bleeding, taking half a gallon of blood, and give another drench: at night, offer him some bran or oats, scalded with sassafras tea, and if it can be procured, let him have green food, fresh from the field, for it has the happy effect of opening the bowels, and cooling the system. His feet should be nicely cleansed out, and stuffed with fresh cow manure; his drink should be at least one-half sassafras tea, with a small handful of salt thrown in. By the morning, should the horse be better, nothing further is necessary, than to be careful not to over-feed him. But should there be no change for the better, tie a small cord just above his knees, and with a lancet or fleam bleed him in a vein that runs around the coronet, just above the hoof. Take from each leg a pint of blood; give a pound of salts, dissolved in three half-pints of water, in form of a drench; keep his feet stuffed with fresh cow manure, and bathe his legs with equal parts of sharp vinegar, spirits, and sweet-oil or lard. By attention to these directions, in two or three days the horse will again be fit for use.

FOUNDER IN HORSES, NO. III.

When a horse is slightly foundered, take a gill of spirits of turpentine, and one pint of whiskey, and drench him with it: when he sweats, rub him down well, and nothing more will be required. For a severe founder, drench him with a quart of melted lard, which is said to be an effectual cure.

FOUNDER IN HORSES, NO. IV.

As soon as you find your horse is foundered, bleed him in the neck, in proportion to the greatness of the founder. In extreme cases you may bleed him as long as he can stand up. Then give him a strong drench of salt and water. Be careful not to let him drink too much water afterwards. Then anoint around the edges of his hoofs with spirits of turpentine, and your horse will be well in one hour.

FOUNDER IN HORSES, NO. V.

If your horse founders over-night, in the morning take a pint of hog's lard, put it in a vessel, and make it boiling hot; clean his hoofs well, and set his foot in the lard. Heat it for each foot, boiling hot; take a spoon and put the fat over the hoof, as near the hair as possible, and if this be done early in the morning he will be fit for use in three hours after. It is better to remove the horse's shoes.

MALANDERS ON HORSES.

This disease consists in chaps, or cracks on the inside of the fore leg, against the knee, discharging a red, sharp humor. To cure it, wash the cracks with warm soap-suds, or old wine; then rub them twice a day with an ointment of hog's lard, mixed with two drachms sublimate of mercury; or apply a poultice of the roots of marsh-mallows and flax-seed, softened with linseed oil, tying it on with a roller. Continue that till the seeds fall off, and the sores become clean; afterwards a mixture of turpentine and quicksilver will be a proper application.

REMEDY FOR THE HEAVES IN HORSES.

Take half a pound of good ginger for a horse; give two tablespoonsful a day; one in the morning and the other in the evening, mixed with wheat bran.

CURE FOR COUGH IN HORSES.

Half a pound of niter, a quarter of a pound of black regulus of antimony, and two ounces of antimony; mix well in a mortar, and make it up into doses of one ounce each; give the horse one dose in a cold mash, every night in mild weather, for three nights. Then omit it for a week. If he does not get better of his cough, repeat it. Care is necessary that the animal should not be exposed while warm, to stand in a cold wind; exercise him gently, and treat him otherwise as usual.

A BROKEN-WINDED HORSE, NO. I.

It is easy to discover a broken-winded horse. By giving him a little brisk exercise he will draw up his flanks, and drop them suddenly, breathe with great difficulty, and make a disagreeable wheezing noise. The seat of the disease appears, from dissection, to be in the lungs; the heart and lungs being found of twice their natural size, which prevents their performing their office with ease, in the action of respiration. Broken wind is sometimes produced in a horse by excessive fatigue, heavy draughts, sudden changes from heat to cold, and other obvious causes. It would be advisable to dispose of such horses at any price, as they are not worth their feeding. This complaint, I believe, does not admit of a perfect cure; but by much care it may be greatly relieved. The food should be compact and nutritious, such as corn and old hay. Carrots are excellent in this case, also parsnips and beets, probably on account of the saccharine matter they contain. Molasses has been given in the water (which should be in very small quantities), with very great success. Some have used tar-water, others prefer the effects of lime-water; but the greatest dependence should be in very sparing supplies of substantial food. The exercise should be regular, but never beyond a walking pace. If the symptomatic cough be troublesome, take away about three quarts of blood every other day.

A BROKEN-WINDED HORSE, NO. II.

This disorder is caused by over-feeding, by violent exercise when the horse is too full, or by letting a horse go into water when he is hot and perspiring; or, it frequently originates from an obstinate cold, not well cured. The only remedy we have known to prove efficient, is to feed a horse on good, healthy food — corn, and not much hay, or feed him upon potatoes, and whenever water is given him, impregnate it with saltpeter and sal-ammoniac. Lime-water, freely given, has in many instances cured this complaint.

THUMPS IN HORSES.

Thumps are caused by over-heating and fast riding or driving. Take one pint of brandy or good whiskey, beat up a quarter of a pound of black pepper, mix it, and drench him. Or take a dozen eggs, hold up his head, and break them, and put them down his throat, shell and all, and he will recover immediately.

WIND GALLS.

Wind galls are spongy and flatulent humors, that make their appearance on both sides of the legs, just above the pastern-joint or fetlock. It is seldom that a horse is found entirely clear of them, particularly about the hind legs, if he be much used.

They are produced by hard usage, strains, bruises, &c., of the back, sinews, or the sheath that covers them, which, by being over-stretched, have some of their fibres ruptured: whence may ooze out the fluid which is commonly found with the included air.

When wind galls make their first appearance, they are easily cured by a bath and bandage. Boil red-oak bark to a strong decoction, add some sharp vinegar, and a little alum, let the parts be fomented twice a day, warm as the hand can be held in it; then take a woollen cloth, dip it in the bath, and bind the ankle up as tightly as possible, without giving pain to the horse.

Should this method not succeed, after a thorough trial, the swelled or puffed parts may be opened with a sharp knife; but blistering with flies is less dangerous, and generally attended with equal success.

Wind galls give to a horse a gouty and clumsy appearance; but I have never known lameness produced by them, or any other injury, except that of stiffening his legs as he advances in years. They furnish strong proof that the animal has rendered much service.

SITFAST ON HORSES.

Sitfast proceeds from the part being frequently bruised with a saddle, until it becomes extremely hard, and after remaining some length of time, is not unlike a horny substance. A cure cannot be performed unless the knife is used for the purpose of cutting it entirely out, after which the fresh wound can be healed with the greatest ease, in a very short time, by using either of the following mixtures:—

1. Take of brandy, half a pint; honey, half a pint; alum, two ounces.

2. Take of blue stone, a quarter of an ounce; spirits of turpentine, two tablespoonsful; spring-water, one pint.

3. Take of sugar of lead, half an ounce; alum, one ounce; copperas, half an ounce. Let the ingredients be well mixed, and the sitfast washed twice a day. After the wound is washed, clean with soap and water.

SCRATCHES.

The scratches is a disease which soon places a horse in such a situation as to render him unfit for any kind of service. When it is permitted to run upon a horse for a length of time without any remedy being applied, the ankles and legs swell very much, and lameness is produced in so great a degree that he is scarcely able to move.

The scratches are produced from many different causes, as hard riding, dirty stables, legs left wet at night without being rubbed, standing on his own manure or mud in the stall where he is confined, &c. Although much inflammation may appear, and the disease discover much inveteracy, the cure is not difficult.

Remedies.—No. 1. Remove the horse to a clean stall; with strong soap-suds wash his legs and ankles nicely; clean out his feet; then wash every inflamed part or sore in strong copperas water, twice a day, until the cure is performed. Take half a gallon of blood from the neck-vein, and give a mash twice a week, of one gallon of bran, one teaspoonful of salt-peter, and one tablespoonful of powdered brimstone. Great attention should be paid to the cleanliness of the stable.

No. 2. After the horse is placed in a clean stall, and his legs and ankles nicely washed with warm soap-suds, take of blue stone, one ounce, of alum, four ounces; to which add half a gallon of strong decoction of red-oak bark; stir them together, until the alum and blue stone are dissolved; then wash the cracks, sores, or inflamed parts twice a day, and the cure will be effected in a very short time. Light or green food would be preferable to any other for a horse thus diseased, until the cure is performed.

No. 3. After washing the legs and ankles clean with soap-suds, take flour of sulphur, or powdered brimstone, one tablespoonful; mix them well together, and anoint the sores and parts inflamed twice a day. A horse will get well much sooner when confined in a clean stall, than by running at large.

No. 4. Boil poke-root to a strong decoction, and bathe the ankles twice a day. In all cases, a clean stable will aid you much in making a quick cure of the scratches.

No. 5. Mix white-lead and linseed-oil, in such proportions as will render the application convenient. Two or three applications will effect a cure.

No. 6. For each dose, take a handful of the roots of dwarf-ash, known in some places by the name of "old man's beard;" chop the roots small, put in two quarts of water, and boil down to about half its quantity. Give this dose every other day, until you have given three; then bleed freely in the neck. A small quantity of lard, or neat's-foot oil, may be applied externally, to soften the sore. For a desperate case, the operation should be repeated.

REMEDY FOR THE POLL-EVIL, OR FISTULA IN HORSES.

When the swelling breaks, or if it has been some time a running sore, it will have a pipe or tube, from which the matter discharges; into this crowd a lump of pearlash, or potash, as large as you can, with your finger. Three such applications will cure the worst case.

ANOTHER REMEDY.

From a horse's rubbing and sometimes striking his poll against the lower edge of the manger, or hanging back in the stall, and bruising the part with the halter, or from the frequent and painful stretchings of the ligaments and muscles, by unnecessary tight reigning, and occasionally, we fear, from a violent blow on the poll, carelessly or wantonly inflicted, inflammation comes on, and a swelling appears — hot, tender, and painful. The first thing to be attempted, is to abate the inflammation by bleeding, physic, and the application of cold lotions to the part; by these means the tumor will sometimes be dispersed. This system, however, must not be pursued too far. If the swelling increases, and the heat and tenderness likewise increase, matter will form in the tumor; and then our object will be to hasten its formation by warm fomentations, poultices, or stimulating embrocations. As soon as matter is formed, which may be known by the softness of the tumor, and before it has time to spread around and eat into the neighboring parts, it should be evacuated. The openings into the tumor must be so contrived, that all the matter shall run out, and continue to run out as it is formed, and not collect at the bottom of the ulcer, irritating and corroding it. This can be effected by a seton alone. The needle should enter at the top of the tumor, penetrate through its bottom, and be brought out at the side of the neck, a little below the abscess. Nothing more than this is needed, except frequent fomentations with warm water, to keep the part clean, and to obviate inflammation. Poll-evil, in its early stage, will frequently be cured. If the ulcer has deepened and spread, and threatens to eat into the ligaments of the joints of the neck, it may be necessary to stimulate its surface, and perhaps painfully so, in order to bring it to a healthy state, and dispose it to fill up; and in extreme cases, even the scalding mixture of the farrier may be called into requisition. This, however, will be ineffectual, except the pus or matter is enabled, by the use of setons, perfectly to run out of the wound; and the application of these setons will require the skill and anatomical knowledge of the veterinary surgeon. In very desperate cases, the wound may not be fairly exposed to the action of our caustic applications, without the division of the ligament of the neck, by which the head is almost entirely supported. This, however, may be done with perfect safety, for although the ligament is carried on to the occipital bone, and some strength is gained by this prolongation of it, the main strength is on the second bone; and the head will continue to be supported, although the ligament should be divided between the second bone and the head. The divided ligament will soon unite again, and its former usefulness will be restored when the wound is healed.

CURE FOR STAGGERS, NO. I.

Take one quart of brandy, or whiskey, and dissolve one ounce of camphor in it, and give for a dose one gill. In about two hours after taking this preparation, the horse will get up. Care should be taken to prevent him from drinking water for twenty-four hours, in which time a complete cure will be effected in nine cases out of ten.

CURE FOR STAGGERS, NO. II.

Symptoms.—The symptoms of the staggers are a drowsiness, eyes inflamed, half shut, and full of tears; the appetite bad; the disposition to sleep generally increased, feebleness, a continual hanging of the head, or resting it on the manger; rearing, falling, and being in a state of insensibility; walking a small circle for a considerable length of time; the ears hot, with a burning fever, &c.

Remedy.—Take from the neck-vein half a gallon of blood, three times a week; take of sassafras tea, three half-pints; plantain juice, half a pint; assafœtida, half an ounce; saltpeter, one teaspoonful. Mix, and give the horse a drink three mornings in a week. Give an injection, composed of one pint of meal, two quarts of water, one quart of molasses, and one spoonful of hog's lard. Let the horse be moderately exercised; and whenever he is standing, he should be well rubbed. Give a mash twice a week, composed of one gallon of bran, one tablespoonful of sulphur, one teaspoonful of saltpeter, one quart of boiling sassafras tea, and an eighth of an ounce of assafœtida, not permitting the horse to drink cold water for six hours afterwards. Should he be much mended by this treatment, nothing more will be necessary, except feeding him on bran, or light food of any kind; but should he appear to receive no benefit from these attentions, in four or five days, take of calomel, twenty-five grains; of opium, two drachms; of camphor, two drachms; powdered fennel-seed, one drachm; of syrup of any kind, a sufficient quantity to make the ingredients into a ball, which may be given every morning for four or five days, by which time the horse will get well, if his disease will admit of cure.

Horses that are confined in the stable never have the staggers; consequently it would be advisable for every person whose situation will admit of it to confine his horses, particularly at night, during the spring and fall months.

BLIND STAGGERS.

This disease appears to be a compression upon the brain, caused by a collection of wind and matter in the forehead. The writer witnessed a cure effected in the following manner: — A hole was bored with a nail gimlet through the skull, on the curl of hair between the eyes. In various instances he has heard of its being tried with uniform success. This remedy was discovered by an attempt to kill, and thus relieve a horse from the distress of this disease. His skull was fractured by the stroke of an axe. The morning following, the horse was found feeding, apparently well. The remedy may be applied by any person, as the horse very soon becomes helpless after the attack, and immediate relief is afforded by letting out the matter, &c.

Those who are too timid to try the above remedy, may resort to one less severe; and as the writer has understood, from a credible source, equally successful. Make a vertical incision in the skin between the eyes; separate it from the skull, so as to make a sufficient cavity to contain a gill of salt, which put in and make it secure. A cure very soon will be effected.

FISTULA.

The fistula in the withers generally proceeds from some blow or bruise, and is the most disagreeable disease to which a horse is subject. I would recommend to every person whose situation will admit of the sacrifice, to dispose of a horse thus unfortunately affected, for whatever sum he would bring, or even give him away, sooner than be at the expense and trouble, and run a risk of performing a cure, which, if completed, would be tedious, and the horse much lessened in value, in consequence of being disfigured by the scar which will unavoidably be left. The remedy here recommended is severe, but it will have the desired effect more speedily than any other.

As soon as the fistula assumes a formidable appearance, fomentations of bitter herbs should be employed, such as wormwood, camomile, bay leaves, mullen, life everlasting, &c., boiled in water to a strong decoction, and, after being strained, should be applied as hot as the horse can bear it without giving pain, by means of large woollen cloths. This application promotes suppuration; and when matter is formed, let the tumor be opened, so that its contents may be completely evacuated; after which, let the sore be nicely washed with strong soap-suds, and apply the following ointment once a day: — Take of verdigris, half an ounce; oil of turpentine, one ounce; copperas, half an ounce; ointment of yellow resin, four ounces; to be well mixed together. As soon as healthy matter is discharged from the fistula, the ointment may be discontinued, and nothing more will be necessary, except keeping it perfectly clean with soap-suds.

When the fistula first makes its appearance, it may be removed or prevented by placing a rowel or seton in each shoulder, just below the swelled or inflamed part. It should be kept running two or three weeks.

FARCY.

To effect a cure in this distressing disease, in its first stage, bleed three times the first week, taking half a gallon of blood at each bleeding; feed principally on bran, oats, or any food easily digested, and the long food green, if to be had. Remove all filth from, or about the stable, taking care to keep it neat and clean afterward. Give three mashes a week, of bran, scalded with sassafras tea, one tablespoonful of powdered brimstone, and one teaspoonful of saltpeter (not permitting the horse to drink for six hours afterward); take half an ounce of assafœtida; wrap it in a clean linen rag, and nail it in the bottom of the manger in which he is fed. All his drink must be equal quantities of sassafras, boiled in water to a strong decoction, and half an ounce of assafœtida should be placed in his watering bucket, in the same manner as directed for the manger. The buds or ulcers should be washed once a day with blue stone, or copperas water; and if the knees or ankles are swelled, spread on a piece of buckskin, mercurial ointment, and bind them up as tight as possible without giving pain.

The second week bleed twice, taking half a gallon of blood each bleeding, if the horse is in tolerable order; or if poor, only half the quantity: give the same number of mashes as directed for the first week; also the same drink, taking care to renew the assafœtida in the manger and bucket, should it be sufficiently exhausted to require it.

The third week bleed but once, taking one quart of blood: in other respects observe the same treatment as directed for the first and second weeks. The horse should be moderately exercised about a mile twice a day, and occasionally should be offered a little hominy, as a change to keep up his appetite. By the time your attentions for the third week expire, if the disease is merely local, it will not only be removed, but the plight of the horse will be much improved.

When the farcy begins to make its appearance epidemically, the case is rendered difficult, and will require the aid of more active medicine. Prepare and give to a horse thus diseased a ball every night for a week, composed of twenty-five grains of calomel, a quarter of an ounce of powdered fennel-seed, a small quantity of syrup of any kind, and as much crumb of loaf-bread as will make a ball about the size of an English walnut.

All buds or ulcers should be washed clean in bluestone water; after which they should be well rubbed around with mercurial ointment once a day; a narrow pitch plaster should be laid on at the joining of the head and neck, in the direction of the throat-latch, for the purpose of taking off the hair, which will happen in two or three days; after which, a lump of mercurial ointment, about the size of a hickory-nut, must be rubbed on the naked part (every night and morning, until the expiration of the week), among the large glands of the throat, until it is entirely absorbed. Added to which, the treatment generally may be the same as before recommended in the more simple stage of the farcy, with these exceptions: the drink should never be cold, but milk-warm; the mashes without sulphur counteract the effects of the calomel and ointment: he should not be bled, and great care should be used to prevent his getting wet, and catching cold in any way, while under the course of physic.

At the expiration of the week, stop the balls and ointment for a week, adding sulphur to the mashes, as directed in the first stage of farcy. At the expiration of the second week, stop the sulphur, and again commence with the balls and ointment. Go on in this manner, continuing to change the medicine each week, until the cure is performed.

It may sometimes happen that a horse's mouth will become sore before the expiration of a week, when taking the balls and using the ointment. Whenever this is discovered, stop with balls, and add sulphur to the mashes, which will readily remove the soreness about the mouth.

STRAINS.

Strains, in whatever part of the horse, either produced from running, slips, blows, or hard riding, are the relaxing, over-stretching or breaking the muscles or tendinous fibres. A strain, unless uncommonly bad, may be cured in a short time by applying the following remedies:

No. 1. Take of sharp vinegar, one pint; spirits of any kind, half a pint; camphor, one ounce; mix them well together, and bathe the part injured twice a day; a piece of flannel, wet with the mixture, and wrapped around the part, will be very beneficial; take from the neck-vein half a gallon of blood.

No. 2. Take of opodeldoc, a piece the size of a marble, and rub it on the strained part with the naked hand twice a day until the hand becomes dry. Should the injured part resist both of these remedies, you may conclude the injury is a very serious one, which nothing but time can relieve, and the horse must be turned out upon grass a sufficient length of time for nature herself to perform the great operation.

RING BONE.

The ring bone partakes of the nature of the spavin, and frequently proceeds from the same cause. It makes its appearance on the lower part of the pastern, and sometimes immediately beyond the coffin-joint. It is a hard and bony substance, and generally reaches half round the ankle, which gives to the ankle an unnatural appearance, and causes the horse to go stiff and lame. Its name has proceeded from its resemblance to a ring. It seldom admits of a cure, consequently a horse diseased with it is worth but little. When the ring bone first makes its appearance, blisters of flies have sometimes been employed with success. But after growing to full size, and remaining some length of time, a cure is hopeless.

Remedy.—A strong preparation of corrosive sublimate added to Spanish flies and Venice turpentine, and mixed with hog's lard, will often dissolve a ring bone.

TO CURE RING HOOF IN HORSES.

Cleanse the sore well with soap and water; wipe dry, and wash with the following mixture twice a day:—Dissolve fifteen grains of corrosive sublimate in six ounces of alcohol; shake well, and it is ready for use.

SPLINT.

The splint is a hard lump or excrescence that grows upon the fore-legs of a horse, between the fetlock and the knee. It is unpleasant to the eye, but seldom does injury, unless situated on the back of the leg, and immediately under the large tendons, in which case lameness is always produced, and the cure rendered difficult.

When the splint is situated in the usual place, and grows so large as to be unfavorable to beauty, bathe the part with hot vinegar twice a day, and rub the knot or splint with a smooth round stick, after bathing for ten or fifteen minutes; by the expiration of a week the knot will perceptibly decrease in size, and finally in a short time will disappear; but should such means not have the desired effect, shave off the hair over the lump, and apply a blister of Spanish flies, which in a short time will effectually remove it. The splint, when first making its appearance, will cause a horse to limp a little; and, as he advances in years, may stiffen him, and cause him to stumble.

STRINGHALT.

The stringhalt affects horses in their hind legs, and consists in a false action or involuntary use of a muscle which twitches one of the legs almost up to the belly; and sometimes the string halt is produced by a muscle being overstrained, or by a violent blow on the hind parts. Good rubbing, and baths of warm vinegar and sweet-oil, afford momentary relief, but a permanent cure need not be expected. A horse thus injured is incapable of faithfully performing a journey, although he may be ridden four or five miles without manifesting excessive fatigue.

SPAVIN.

A spavined horse may be considered as one completely ruined; for a permanent cure can rarely be effected, if attempted even on its first appearance.

The spavin is a lump, knot, or swelling, on the inside of the hock, below the joint, that benumbs the limbs, and destroys the free use of the hind legs. It causes a horse to be extremely lame, and to experience, apparently, very excruciating pain.

In the purchase of a horse, great respect should be paid to his bringing up his hind parts well, as a spavined horse never makes a full step with the leg affected; also to the shape of his hocks, in order to discover if there is any knot or unnatural prominence about the joints, which is an evidence of the spavin. When a horse is thus diseased, he is unfit for any kind of service, even the meanest drudgery, being in constant pain, and unable to perform labor. Horses sometimes have the spavin when there is no lump apparent near the joint, the disease being seated in the joint. To detect such spavin, have the horse ridden in three quarters speed, about one mile out and back, occasionally fretting, cracking, and drawing him up suddenly and short; after which, let him be ridden in cold water up to the belly: then place him in a stall, without interruption, for about half an hour, by which time he will be perfectly cool. Then have him led out, and moved gently. If he has received a temporary cure of spavin, he will show lameness. A blister of Spanish flies applied to the part affected (after shaving off the hair), with a bath of strong spirits or vinegar, and a week's rest, will frequently suspend the lameness produced by the spavin for a time; but a radical cure may not be expected.

ANOTHER REMEDY.

The following has been found to cure a bone spavin in its first stages, when properly applied. Add to two tablespoonsful of melted lard, one of cantharides, made fine or pulverized, and a lump of corrosive sublimate, as large as a pea, pulverized — all melted up together, and applied once a day till used up. This quantity is for one leg, and may be relied on as a cure. It will make a sore, and the joint will be much weakened while applying the medicine, but no need of alarm; it will be all right when healed up.

GLANDERS.

As an experiment, where the usual remedies had failed, a strong decoction of tobacco-juice was given internally, and proved successful.

BIG HEAD IN HORSES.

The following treatment has been tried and found to afford temporary relief: — The duct that passes from the eye to the nose was laid bare, or an incision made in the large part of the nose, and the wound burned with a hot iron. But the horse, about two years afterwards, became diseased, dwindled away, and lost, measurably, the use of the parts. Afterwards, the following experiment on the same horse proved highly successful: — He was thrown and tied; then a hot iron run through his head, inserting it into the lump on one side, and carrying it through the lump upon the other. The horse in a short time was well, and never after had any symptoms of the disease. Others were treated in the same way, with equal success.

LAMPASS.

All young horses are subject to the lampass, and some suffer extremely before it is discovered.

It is a swelling or enlarging of the gums on the inside of the upper jaw; the growth is sometimes so large as to prevent a horse from eating with any comfort. The remedy is simple, and after being applied, a horse will improve in his condition with great rapidity.

Take a hot iron, flat, sharp, and a little crooked at the end, burn the lampass out just below the level of the teeth, using great care to prevent the hot iron from bearing or resting on the teeth. After the operation is performed, the horse should be given a little bran or meal, with a small quantity of salt in it. Some farriers have recommended cutting for the lampass, which only gives momentary relief, and would require the same operation to be performed every three or four months; but when it is once burned out, it never again makes its appearance.

HOOKS OR HAWS.

The hooks or haws in a horse is the growing of a horny substance upon the inner edge of the washer or caruncle of the eye, which may be found in the inner corner, next to the nose. When this disease makes its appearance, the washer or caruncle is enlarged with great rapidity, and the ligament that runs along the edge of this membrane becomes extremely hard, or like a cartilage; and whenever it arises to this state, it draws, compresses, and causes great pain to the eyes, produces a tightness of the skin, a stiffness of the hind legs, and finally a general spasmodic affection, throughout the whole system.

The eyes are often inflamed, and sometimes diseased, without their having the hooks. For the purpose of ascertaining the fact, take hold of the bridle, and raise the horse's head as high as you can, with convenience, reach: if he is diseased with the hooks, the washer or caruncle of the eye, while his head is raised up, will cover at least one-half the surface of the eye-ball. When this is the case, take a common sized needle, with a strong thread [having placed on the horse's nose a twitch, to prevent his moving]; then take in your thumb and finger the washer or caruncle of the eye, and pass the needle through it, about a quarter of an inch from the outer edge, and inside the horny substance; draw it gently with the needle and thread, until you have a fair chance of performing the operation; then with a sharp knife cut the piece out taken with the needle, which must not be larger than one-fourth the size of a half-dime: wash the eyes for two or three mornings with salt and water, bathe his legs up to his belly in equal parts of warm vinegar, spirits, and oil, or fresh butter, and give a mash of one and a half gallons of bran or oats, one tablespoonful of flour of sulphur, one teaspoonful of saltpeter, and the cure will be performed, in all probability, in four or five days. Great care should be taken not to cut too large a piece from the caruncle, as it disfigures the eye, and sometimes produces blindness.

LOCKJAW.

The lockjaw being so fatal in its consequences, it is a fortunate circumstance that it occurs so seldom among horses.

It commences with a difficulty in mastication; and shortly after the jaws are so completely and immovably closed, that it is with much difficulty that medicine can be administered. The muscles of the neck appear to be much contracted, and the animal seems to suffer great pain.

The lockjaw is frequently brought on by trifling causes, such as cuts, wounding of nerves, tendons, &c. Generally speaking, the cure is uncertain; but it will chiefly depend on opium, the warm bath, and other anti-spasmodics. Sometimes the sudden application of cold water, in great quantities, has been serviceable; friction of turpentine, oil, or spirits, generally proves useful, as does a clyster made with two ounces of spirits of hartshorn, four ounces of oil of turpentine, and the yolk of three or four eggs, mixed with a quart of strong ale and gin, or whiskey. It is a great object to promote urine, sweat, &c. Opium, camphor, and copious bleedings have been found, in some cases, very beneficial; and when they have failed, hartshorn, ether, opium, and brandy, have been employed with some success; though the lockjaw is often a symptom of approaching dissolution, and frequently defies the power of all kinds of medicine that have yet been employed in its treatment.

GRAVEL IN THE HOOFS.

The gravel in the hoof is an incident that happens to horses in traveling, and is brought on by small stones or grit getting between the hoof and shoe, settling to the quick, and then inflaming and festering; it produces lameness, and causes a horse to undergo very excruciating pain. The first step necessary for a horse's relief is to have his shoes taken off and get the stones out. You may readily determine where they lie, by pressing the edge of the hoof with a pair of pincers, after all the gravel is removed, which may be known by a discontinuation of the blackness of the place. The wound caused by cutting for the gravel may be easily healed by melting together equal parts of beeswax, resin, fresh butter, or sweet-oil, and pouring the mixture on the wound, warm as the animal can bear it without giving pain. Then warm a little tar or pitch, and pour a small quantity over the wound and its neighboring parts to keep out the dust and defend the foot from any hard substance for a few days, by which time it will get well.

STONE OR GRAVEL IN THE BLADDER.

Fortunately the stone is a disease not very common among horses; but whenever it makes its appearance, unless some remedy is immediately employed, its consequences are to be much dreaded. It consists in small gravel or stones being lodged in the bladder, which prevent a free discharge of urine, and produce the most excruciating pain. The horse will linger and pine away until he can scarcely support the burden of life.

Symptoms.—Frequent stretching, groaning, and many fruitless attempts to pass water, which will finally be discharged by a few drops at a time, with great apparent pain, a shrinking of the flesh, although the appetite is good, no fever, but a dull, sluggish, and sleepy appearance, wanting much in his usual spirits.

Remedy.—Take of marsh-mallows, water-melon seed, and asparagus, each two large handsful; boil them in three quarts of water to one quart, and add one teaspoonful of saltpeter, and give the whole as a drench, after being nicely strained.

Take of sweet-oil, or fresh butter, one tablespoonful; grease his sheath, and draw out gently and grease his penis; also grease the large seam from the penis up near the anus; and with the hand, bearing a little, stroke the seam downward to the end of the penis, for ten minutes every hour, until the horse has a urinary discharge, which in all probability will take place in one or two hours after taking the drench. Should some blood be passed, it may be no cause of alarm, and will clearly prove there is gravel in the urinary passages. Repeat the dose in three hours, should the desired effect not be produced.

HIDE-BOUND.

A horse is said to be hide-bound when his skin will not slip under the pressure of the hand, but sticks as fast to the ribs as if it were glued.

Horses are sometimes hide-bound in consequence of some violent disease, and it is often a bad symptom; but, generally, this tightness of the skin proceeds from bad or insufficient provender, cruel usage, and sometimes from worms.

The first thing necessary for performing a cure is to offer better treatment to the animal, giving him plenty of light food, such as bran, oats, &c., and a clean stable, with fresh litter. Then take from the neck-vein half a gallon of blood. At night give a mash composed of one gallon of bran, scalded with sassafras tea, one tablespoonful of flour of sulphur, or powdered brimstone, and one teaspoonful of saltpeter, not permitting him to drink for six hours afterward. On the second day, at twelve o'clock, take of copperas, two tablespoonsful; of warm sassafras tea, one quart; saltpeter, one teaspoonful. Mix, and give them as a drench. Have the horse well rubbed, and in a few days he will be entirely relieved.

YELLOW WATER.

The yellow water is very infectious. It is extremely fatal in its consequences, unless some remedy is employed shortly after it makes its appearance.

Symptoms of Yellow Water.—The characteristics of this disease are a dusky yellowness of the eyes, lips, and bars of the mouth; a dull, sluggish appearance, a loss of appetite; the excrement hard, dry, yellow, and sometimes of a pale or light green; the urine uncommonly dark, of a dirty brown color, and when discharged a length of time has the appearance of blood.

Remedy.—Take of assafœtida, one ounce; camphorated spirits, four tablespoonsful; warm water, one pint. Mix, and give them as a drench, for three or four mornings successively. Take of bran, one and a half gallons; flour of sulphur, one tablespoonful; antimony, twenty grains. Mix them well together, and with a strong decoction of sassafras, scald the bran, forming a mash, which must be given three nights in the week, not permitting the horse to get wet, or drink water, except it is milk-warm. His stable should be a comfortable one, and he should have a clean bed of straw placed under him. Bleed twice in the neck-vein, taking half a gallon of blood at each bleeding, within the week. Let his exercise be regular and moderate; and by the expiration of nine or ten days, the cure, in all probability, will be performed.

REMEDY FOR THE BOTTS, NO. I.

A tablespoonful of slacked lime, given three times a week, in bread mashes, for near two weeks, has caused the botts to pass off in quantities, varying from ten to twenty during the night.

As an evidence of its good effects, a gentleman who has tried it in many cases, says he has not lost a horse since he began to use it. A large number of the botts thus expelled had the appearance of being dead. This fact induced him to put some of the live ones in a strong solution of lime-water (spirits of turpentine having produced no effect on them), and all those put into lime-water were dead in eight-and-forty hours.

Lime-water is a certain preventive in keeping cattle from taking the murrain. As an evidence of this fact, it has been used among cattle three times per week, mixed with salt, for three or four years; and in that time not a single cow, or steer, or ox, was lost by this disease. In the mean time, some of the neighbors lost nearly all the cattle they owned.

No doubt it is a sure and infallible remedy for botts in horses, and a preventive of murrain among cattle.

REMEDY FOR THE BOTTS, NO. II.

To make botts let go their hold, give the horse a quantity of molasses or dissolved sugar, with a quart of sweet milk; in thirty minutes, you will find the horse at ease. Then pulverize an eighth of a pound of alum, dissolved in a quart of warm water, and drench your horse. After two hours, or less, give the horse one pound of salts, and you will find the botts in the dung. The molasses and sweet milk will cause the botts to let go, and prey upon the sweetening. The alum contracts them, and the salts pass them off.

REMEDY FOR THE BOTTS, NO. III.

The ingredients are simple, and too mild to produce any injurious effects on the animal to which they may be administered. They consist of new milk, honey, or molasses, common salt and water, and linseed-oil. The manner of preparing and administering is as follows: — As soon as the disease (the symptoms of which are unerring) is ascertained, drench the horse, fasting if possible, with a quart of fresh milk saturated with honey, molasses, or sugar; to be preferred in the order stated. Leave him at rest for two hours; at the expiration of which, having previously prepared some strong brine, by boiling as much common salt as can be dissolved in it, drench him as before with a pint of it when cool. After a similar period of two hours, give him half a pint of linseed-oil, and the remedy is complete.

TO KILL LICE ON HORSES, COWS AND HOGS.

Take the water in which potatoes have been boiled, rub it all over the skin. The lice will be dead within two hours, and never will multiply again.

DISTEMPER IN CATTLE

May be cured by boiling the common poke-root to a strong decoction, and administering a quart of it three times a day.

DISEASES AND TREATMENT OF CATTLE.

All cattle brought to the South from England, as well as those from the North and West, are very liable to be attacked with a fatal disease, similar to an inflammation of the brain.

Young cattle, from eight months to one year old, are less subject to it than those more advanced in life. If they survive the summer and autumn, I consider them safe, although great care should be taken of them the second season. They should be brought as early in the fall as possible, kept in good growing condition through the winter, and in the spring be removed to a high, healthy position, have easy access to pure water, and their pasture as much shaded as the nature of the ground will admit. In August and September, they should be kept in a cool stable, during the heat of the day, and at night also, the dew at that season being almost as injurious as the intense heat of the sun.

With these precautions, probably more than half would escape the disease, the first indication of which is usually a languid appearance of the animal, followed by the loss of appetite, short, quick breathing, with more or less fever, and not unfrequently a cough.

I have hitherto considered this disease, when once established, incurable. I have recently learned, however, that by sawing off the horns, close to the head, nine out of ten would recover. They may be bled copiously, which relieves the dullness about the eyes. After the bleeding is stopped, bind cloths, plastered with tar, around the stump, as a protection against flies.

TO KILL LICE ON CATTLE.

We have been informed by a gentleman who has for many years kept a large stock of cattle, that fine, dry sand scattered on the back, neck, and sides of the animals, is an effectual remedy against these vermin. He collects dry sand, and puts it in a box or tub in the barn, and occasionally applies it during the winter, by sifting or strewing it over the body of each creature, with complete success in ridding it of its troublesome guests.

ANOTHER REMEDY.

Make a strong sassafras tea, or red pepper tea (or a mixture of both is preferable), with a reasonable portion of lard, and rub or wash the animal with it every two or three days. It will kill the lice, and destroy the nits as fast as they hatch; and, by a few washings, the animal will soon be rid of the lice. It is a sure and safe remedy.

TO DESTROY VERMIN ON CATTLE.

A strong decoction of tobacco, washed over a beast infected with vermin, will generally drive them away. It sometimes will make the beast very sick for a short time. But a better remedy is to mix plenty of strong Scotch snuff in train oil, and rub the back and neck of the creature with it. This will effectually kill or drive away all vermin from a quadruped.

TO DESTROY VERMIN ON CATTLE, AND CURE THE MANGE.

Put into an earthen vessel four ounces of flour of sulphur, and a pound weight of nut-oil; place the vessel upon a moderate fire, and stir the mixture with a piece of wood, until part of the flour of sulphur is dissolved, and the oil has acquired a reddish-brown color; then remove it from off the fire; and before it is entirely cold, add four ounces of essence of turpentine; then stir it again, until it is incorporated. This preparation is neither expensive nor compli cated; and when used, is merely put upon the parts infected with a feather.

HORN DISTEMPER, OR HORN AIL,

Is a disorder incident to horned cattle, by which the internal substance of the horn (commonly called the pith, which is the spongy part of the bone), wastes away, &c. This disorder may be known by a dullness in the countenance, a sluggish motion, want of appetite, a desire to lie down frequently, shaking the head, and appearing dizzy, &c. To be sure of this disease, take a small gimlet, and perforate the horn two or three inches above the head: if it is hollow, and no blood follows, it is the hollow horn. This distemper is generally brought on by poor keeping, &c.

Bore each horn at the upper and lower side, that the drain may have vent, and administer at least two or three doses of salts, or some gentle purgative; inject into the horn strong vinegar. This will cleanse the horn, and effect a cure. Sawing off the horn is sometimes resorted to, but the above treatment is preferable.

ON THE DISEASE COMMONLY CALLED THE HOLLOW HORN.

This is a disease that is highly inflammatory and infectious, and the animal having it ought to be removed from the herd until well.

The following mode of treatment has been found very successful, and the beast is soon restored to a thriving state. As soon as you discover an animal affected with the hollow horn, bleed it from the neck (in the same vein in which a horse is bled), from two to six or seven quarts, according to its age, size, and condition, and administer three quarters to one pound and a half of glauber salts; with a middle-sized gimlet, open the horns through and through, marking the holes, that they be perpendicular in the usual position the animal carries its head, so that the pus formed may have a free discharge as soon as the horns are opened; put through the hole into each about a tablespoonful of strong vinegar, in which some salt and black pepper, ground, has been put. The day following, the horns must be again opened, and cleansed from the pus, which generally is now formed, and about half a teaspoonful of spirits of turpentine put into each horn; and a little on the poll of the animal daily, during the continuance of the disease. One bleeding is generally sufficient, but there are cases in which it is necessary to repeat it three times, as also the salts. The food, during the continuance of the disease, is important — corn in every shape is bad — potatoes are of great use (with a small quantity of brewer's grains); and the animal ought to have from one to two and a half pecks daily, with hay in the winter, and grass if in the summer. Potatoes have a wonderful effect on the animal, as soon as the bowels are well cleansed; the importance of which any person will be convinced of who observes the discharge of the animal. In some obstinate cases, give daily from a half to one ounce of niter, sprinkled with potatoes. It is important, in the first bleeding, to take as much blood as the animal will bear, as the fever is more easily checked by one large bleeding than two small ones, and the animal better able to bear it. In many cases the bleeding and salts have been sufficient without opening the horns, and when taken in the early stage will generally be found to answer; but the boring certainly assists in forming anew the internal part of the horn, and as soon as it commences forming, the holes in the horn should be allowed to close. An animal having the hollow horn should be sheltered from the inclemency of the weather, during its continuance. No age appears exempt from its attacks. I have seen it in a yearling, as well as at all subsequent ages.

The fleam for bleeding cattle should be rather deeper than that used for a horse, the vein in the neck not lying so near the surface: the orifice is closed with a pin, in the same way as in bleeding a horse.

HOOF-AIL.

Blue vitriol finely pulverized, and applied to the diseased part of the hoof, once a day for two or three days, is all that is necessary to effect a cure. One application is sometimes sufficient.

ANOTHER REMEDY.

This disease is generally brought on by driving cattle on hard or muddy roads. The first symptom is lameness. When this is noticed, the foot on examination will be found to be in some degree inflamed and swollen. Wash the foot in pickle as strong as you can make it. This has frequently proved effectual, but if it does not, an ointment made of corrosive sublimate and hog's lard, rubbed in the slit between the hoofs, is a good remedy. If it be neglected, the parts below the hoof will become dry and horny, in which case the hard part must be cut out, and the wounded flesh cured with healing ointment.

TO RELIEVE CHOKED CATTLE.

After an ineffectual resort to the usual remedies, a choked ox has been relieved by holding up his head, and pouring into his mouth a strong solution of soap and water. The relief was instantaneous, the turnip with which he was choked passing down immediately.

HOVEN CATTLE.

Have a decoction of anise and fennel-seed prepared by boiling for a few minutes a handful composed of equal quantities of the two, in a pint of water. To this add one pound of hog's lard, and give it to the animal in the usual way. If one dose is not effectual, give a second.

SWELLED OR SNARLED UDDERS IN COWS.

Cows, soon after calving, are subject to have swellings or knots in their udders; this is more particularly the case with heifers with their first calves. It sometimes proceeds from colds contracted prior to calving; at others, from the inability of the calf to extract all the milk, which throws the cow into a feverish condition, and the formation of indurated surfaces consequently follows. Should fever accompany these lumps, a little cooling medicine will be proper, such as a solution of half a pound of Epsom salts in a drench, to be followed with good nourishing messes, say one peck of bran, and half a pound of flaxseed-meal, to be first boiled, and given warm, morning and night, for a few days. To reduce the swelling in the udder, the following receipt will be found excellent:—

Take a handful of rue, and the same quantity of wormseed; bruise them both well, and put them into a skillet or other vessel, with a pound of unsalted butter, fresh from the churn; simmer the whole well over a slow fire for an hour; then strain the mixture through a sieve or linen cloth, and you have the best ointment that can be applied. Let the inflamed and hardened part be gently anointed three times a day with the hand, and in a few days the cure will be effected, if this remedy is applied in time.

Care should always be taken before the calf is turned to the cow, for several days after she has calved, to let the dairy-woman draw off a portion of the milk; by so doing, you are sure the calf will extract the rest: by thus emptying the cow's udders, you will prevent the ill-consequences which ensue, where a part of the milk is left in the bag.

A CURE FOR MURRAIN.

Give one and a half ounces pearlash, dissolved in two quarts of iron-water (from a blacksmith's trough). If not better in five hours, give half an ounce more in one quart of water. The water should be warm. Give no drink but warm water, for two days. Give warm mash to eat.

CURE FOR THE BLOODY MURRAIN.

Take a piece of poke-root, as large as a man's fist, say half a pound in weight, cut it fine, add two quarts of water, boil it down to one quart. This quantity must be given once a day, for two or three days, to a cow or bull, when the cure will be effected.

CURE FOR MURRAIN IN CATTLE.

Glauber salts, one pound; niter and cream of tartar in powder, each one ounce; ginger pulverized, two ounces; treacle or molasses, four teaspoonsful; mix for a dose. If it does not succeed in twenty-four hours, add strained turpentine, four ounces; Armenian bale bayberries, and red-saunders in powder, of each two ounces; mix in a mortar, and beat it into a proper consistence for the bale or ball.

FILMS ON THE EYE.

The easiest, as well as most effectual remedy for removing a film from the eye of an animal, is simply to put a teaspoonful of molasses on the eye-ball. Oxen, horses, cows, and sheep, have, in this manner, been relieved.

SALT FOR CATTLE.

Let it be remembered, that salt, when given to animals, enables the farmer to increase his live stock, and keep them in health: hence it ought freely to be given to sheep, and cattle of every description; but, to imitate nature, it should be previously dissolved, and then mixed with pure, fine clay, in a mass, which is to be placed under a shelter, so that the animals may lap it at pleasure.

A CURE FOR SCOURS IN CALVES.

Take a tablespoonful of finely powdered chalk, and a like quantity of ground ginger, put it in a bowl, pour boiling new milk on it, half a pint; stir it well, and then give this dose about milk warm, night and morning, to the calf, and in nine cases out of ten, two doses will be sufficient.

DISEASES OF CALVES.

The diseases of calves are principally confined to a species of convulsions which now and then attacks them, and which sometimes arise from worms, and at others from cold. When the first cause operates, it is relieved by giving a mild aloetic purge, or in default of that, a mild dose of oil of turpentine, half an ounce, night and morning. In the second, wrap up the animal warm, and drench with ale and laudanum, a drachm. Calves are also subject to diarrhœa, or scouring, which will readily yield to the usual medicines.

CURE FOR POISONED SHEEP.

In the spring of the year, sheep and lambs are very apt to eat the green leaves of the low laurel, or camp-kill, as it is sometimes called. This brings on a retching or vomiting of a greenish fluid, which the sheep again swallow down. The animal begins to swell and becomes stupid, refuses to eat or drink, and finally dies. As soon as a sheep is discovered to be sick, and throw up the fluid above mentioned, fix a gag in its mouth by taking a short stick, or a corn-cob, tying a string at each end, put it into the mouth, and passing the string up over the head of the sheep, so as to keep the gag in, and the mouth open. This prevents them from swallowing. A dose of weak ammonia is very good. Roasted onions put under the fore-legs are also beneficial. A gentleman recommends a strong decoction of the bruised twigs of white-ash, given in doses of two spoonsful to a sheep, especially if administered within the last twenty-four hours after the sheep has eaten the poison.

DISEASES OF SHEEP.

The great losses which wool-growers frequently sustain in consequence of the sickness and death of large numbers of their flocks, have induced us to compile from a rare and valuable English work a synopsis of the diseases to which sheep are liable, together with the symptoms by which they are known, and the treatment by which they are remedied. The causes of the disease are in some cases assigned, and it is believed if they are carefully avoided, and the remedies promptly and faithfully applied, the losses from disease and death will in a great degree be prevented, and the profits arising from their fleeces and young be materially increased. As the remedies are simple, and the ingredients composing the prescriptions within the reach of every farmer, it is to be hoped that every wool-grower who has the misfortune to have a diseased flock will give them a thorough trial.

Fever.—Fever in sheep is an inflamed state of the blood, disordering the eye and mouth, and affecting the whole body, though not visibly. When any of the symptoms of a fever appear, the feet of the sheep should be examined, and if found to be hot, there is no doubt of the character of the disease: other diseases will produce an inflammation of the eyes and mouth, but hot feet are an infallible symptom of fever. This disease is often fatal in itself, and frequently induces others which are equally so. The cause is generally a cold. When only two or three of the flock are affected by it, the case is less desperate; but when many are attacked with it, it is more fatal. The remedy is to keep the sheep in warmer and more sheltered places: bleed and give the following medicine:—

Heat a quart of ale, and dissolve in it an ounce of nithritate, add half an ounce of Virginia snake-root, and one drachm cochineal in powder. This quantity serves for four doses, and one of them is to be given morning and evening. If the sheep is bound in its body, an ounce of sanative electuary is to be mixed with each dose; but if looser than ordinary, it ought not to be checked.

PURGING.—Leave nature to her course when a purging comes on with a fever; but when the fever is abated, it should be stopped; and the same remedy that answers for this purpose may be adopted for such purgings as come on of themselves. Boil a quarter of a pound of raspings of logwood in two quarts of water till but a quart is left, and when it is nearly boiled down, put in a stick of cinnamon, strain it off, and give the sheep a quarter of a pint, four times a day, till the purging ceases. If this does not produce the desired result, the following addition will render it sure of success:—To every dose, add a quarter of an ounce of diascordium without honey, and ten grains of Japan earth powdered, and give the doses only morning and evening.

TAG.—The tag is an external disease, owing to the complaint last named. It is a distemper of the tail, beginning with filth and foulness, and ending in ulceration. The tag is situated in the inner part of the tail; it consists of scabs and sores, very painful and wasting to the animal and is owing to the fouling of this part by purging; that tag is worst which follows a fever, because the inflamed state of the blood tends to increase the disorder, and when it begins during the continuance of the disease, the matter of the fever may chance to settle it there. Two things are to be done; the first is to stop the purging, and the other to clean the tail. The last mentioned remedy, either in its weaker or stronger form, is to be used to stop the purging; and the tail being clipped, and the sore part laid bare, wash it first with milk and water, blood-warm, and then with lime-water; after this, turn the sheep into a clean, dry pasture. Two days after look at it again, and if not well, repeat the washing, and anoint it with grease and tar mixed together. Twice doing of this is generally sufficient to complete the cure.

Disease of the Lungs. — Sheep are subject to be diseased in the lungs, which is easily perceived by their breathing or by their coughing. Nothing requires a more speedy remedy, for they grow incurable when it is neglected a short time, and die as men with a consumption. Change of their pasture is essential to the cure; without it, no remedy is effectual. It is owing to cold, and generally attacks sheep that have been kept on low grounds in wet weather. When any of the flock exhibit symptoms of diseased lungs, drive them into an enclosed pasture where there is short grass and a gravelly soil, and where there is spring or other running water; bruise a basketful of the leaves of colts-foot, and press out the juice; bruise a quantity of plantain leaves and roots together, and press out the juice; mix these, and bruise as much garlic as will yield about a fourth part as much juice as one of the others; mix all together, and add to them a pound of honey, an ounce of anise-seed, and an ounce and a half of elecampane; give a quarter of a pint of this warm once in a day, to every sheep that is affected, and it will, by degrees, make a perfect cure.

JAUNDICE. — Sheep are more subject than any other animals to obstructions of the liver. When this is the case, it is seen in a yellowness of the eyes, and a tint of the same kind in the skin. Farmers, in some places, call this the choler, or, in their language, the color. When sheep are attacked with jaundice, they should be put into an open pasture, and kept in moderate motion, but not fatigued. Boil, in four gallons of water, two pounds of fennel-roots, the same quantity of parsley-roots, and twice as much of the roots of cough-grass, all cut small. When the water is very strong of them, and there is about half the quantity left, strain it off by pressing it hard; bruise as much great celandine as will yield three pints of juice; add this to the liquor, and put in three drachms of salt of steel; mix all together, and every day beat as much of it as will serve to give each sheep that is ill a gill and a half for a dose. This, with the forementioned directions, rarely fails of a cure.

STOPPAGE IN THE THROAT. — Sheep affected with stoppage in the throat wheeze and breathe with difficulty. It is commonly occasioned by bad pasturage and colds. The remedy is to put them on higher ground; keep them warm, and give them the following medicine: — Bruise a good quantity of pennyroyal, and squeeze out the juice; put to a quart of it a pound of honey, and half a pint of sharp vinegar. Give half a pint of this, blood-warm, every night.

STURDINESS. — This is a giddiness in the head. It is owing, principally, to rich feeding. The remedy is as follows: — Bleed profusely, and add the following treatment: bruise some roots of wild valerian, squeeze out the juice, heat it, and give a quarter of a pint: repeat the dose every four hours. When the sheep is recovered, turn it upon the common, or into some barren, hilly pasture. It will be kept from relapses by having but little food, and that perfectly wholesome. If the disease returns, it is commonly fatal.

WOOD EVIL. — This disease is a kind of cramp; it seizes the legs, and will often attack a whole flock at once. Cold and wet are the cause; lying under the dripping trees in rainy seasons has often occasioned it, and hence its name. In order to effect a cure, the sheep must be removed to a dry pasture, and there proper remedies may take effect. The following medicine is recommended: — Boil in a large quantity of ale, as much cinquefoil, and hedge mustard, as can be well stirred into it. When the liquor is very strong, strain it off, and add a pint of juice of valerian root to every gallon. Give half a pint of this morning and evening. Boil in vinegar a large quantity of the leaves of hedge mustard, and with the hot liquor rub the legs.

STAGGERS.—Sheep, as well as horses, are sometimes afflicted with the staggers. It is occasioned by improper food. Oak leaves and buds are particularly prejudicial. They bind the bowels, and staggers frequently follow. The symptoms are the same as in sturdiness, but more violent, and there is generally a trembling at the same time in all the limbs. To cure this disorder, dissolve half an ounce of assafœtida in two quarts of water; give a quarter of a pint, warm, every three hours. It commonly opens the bowels at the same time that it takes immediate effect on the nervous system, and thus performs a cure. When the sheep are recovered, let them be kept out of the way of a return to the same food, and they will be in no danger of a relapse.

ANOTHER. — Half a pint of hog's lard melted and poured down a sheep, will cure the blind staggers in ten minutes.

SCAB. — This is a disorder to which sheep are very liable. When they are kept in dry, wholesome pastures, they are but seldom afflicted with the scab; but when they are on low, wet grounds, or get under the drippings of trees in bad seasons, they are frequently affected by it in the severest manner. The symptoms are scurvy skins, which in a little time rise to scabs; the wool grows loose, and the sheep pine and become lean. If they are attacked in a season when they can be sheared, it should be immediately done, as nothing is so sure to effect a cure. If the season will not admit of shearing, they must be washed with soap-suds, made very strong, and used warm with a piece of flannel or a brush. After this, they must be let loose into a clean pasture, and driven up again as soon as well dried, and the sore parts of the skin must be well wetted with lime-water. The scurvy part of the skin must be attended to; and the doing this three times, at intervals of two days, will generally effect a cure. But if it fails, the parts that have been thus washed and cleansed must be anointed with a mixture of equal parts of tar and grease, and they will soon be perfectly well. No inward medicines are required, for the complaint is only of the skin.

ANOTHER.—A gentleman informs us, that his flock were so much afflicted with scab, that he lost one hundred, and the value of his fleeces was diminished eleven cents per pound, in consequence of the diseased state of the animals. He cured them of disease, and restored his flock to fine condition, in which they still remain, by the following:—He boiled eight pounds of tobacco in eight pailsful of water, down to five pailsful; to this he added five pailsful of weak ley from wood-ashes, one barrel of soft soap, and some water. Filling in part a half-hogshead with the liquid, he dipped into it three hundred and fifty sheep, liquid being added as required; the sheep, as fast as they were dipped, were placed in another tub, and the liquid pressed out of the fleece with the hands. The wash cleanses the skin from all scurf, kills the lice and ticks, promotes perspiration, and greatly facilitates the growth of the fleece and health of the animal. There is no doubt of the utility of any application that destroys the lice and ticks, and fits the skin, by thoroughly cleansing it, to perform its all-important functions.

RED WATER.—This is an inflammation of the skin that often raises it into blisters, in which is contained a sharp humor, thin, watery, and colored with blood. Nothing should be done to strike it in, but the cure must be effected by correcting the bad state of the blood. Sheep afflicted with it should be separated from the flock, otherwise it will be apt to spread through the whole. They should also be put into a pasture where the grass is sweet, and where they can have access to good water. Mix half an ounce of sulphur with an ounce of honey; work it well together, and then divide it into two parts; dissolve one of these in half a pint of juice of nettles, and give it every day for a fortnight. Slit the blisters when they are full of this watery humor, and having let the matter out, wet the place with juice of wormwood; after four days of this course, bleed them, and then continue the same method till they are well.

Foot Worm.—Sheep are liable to breed worms between their feet, principally, however, when they are kept in wet pastures. It is very painful to them, and will make them pine away. It is perceived by their frequently holding up one foot, and by setting it tenderly down. Let the foot be washed clean, particularly between the toes, and there will be found a little lump, like a tuft of hair; this is the head of the wound. It is to be taken out with care, for it is of a tender substance, and if it be broken in the foot it will occasion inflammation. The best method is to open the flesh on each side of it, and then, by means of a pair of nippers, to take it out. Dress the wound with tar and grease, melted together in equal quantities, and turn the sheep loose. It is better to put them into a fresh pasture; for, if the same disorder returns, it is generally worse.

Wildfire.—This is a violent inflammation, not unlike St. Anthony's fire, upon the skin in different places, and generally affects the whole flock. The following is a method of cure:—Separate such as are affected with the disease from the flock, bleed, and prepare the following external remedy: Bruise the leaves of wild chervil, and add to them as much lime-water as will make the whole very soft; when it is beaten up together, add as much powder of fenugveck seed as will reduce it to pap; then put it into a pan, and set it in a cool place; rub the inflamed part carefully with this every evening, and make as much lie on as can be kept there; it will take effect during the time of rest, and is to be repeated as long as there is occasion.

Disorders of the Eyes.—Sheep are often affected with colds falling upon their eyes, and almost blinding them. The remedy is to press out the juice of great celandine, and drop a quantity of it into the eyes, night and morning.

Dropsy.—Sheep are often swelled with water in their bellies; and this, if not regarded in time, is certain death. There are two parts in which it is lodged; the one is between the outward flesh and the rind, the other within the rind. The first is easily cured; for the other, nothing effectual can be done. The method, in the first case, is by a coarse kind of tapping. An opening is to be made in the flesh, and a quill thrust in. This will give the water a free passage out, and the wound heals of itself. But when the sheep is emaciated, nature will not have strength to heal it; and the sheep must be examined daily, and the wound dressed with tar and grease. It must also be put into a fresh, dry, and wholesome pasture, and then disposed of as soon as recruited; for this is a disorder that never fails to return upon any mismanagement in keeping.

THE ROT. — This is the most destructive disease to which sheep are subject. Like the murrain, it is contagious, and generally spreads through the whole flock, and often over the neighboring country. Flocks that are fed upon open commons are more subject to it than such as have shelter and are taken care of at night. It frequently prevails in cold seasons, and when drizzling rains come on soon after shearing. Want of food will also occasion this disease, as will likewise the eating of such grass as is full of unwholesome plants. These are among the causes of this fatal distemper; but the worst and most common is infection. Keep sheep out of the way of these causes of the rot, and the same care will preserve them from most other disorders to which they are liable; damp grounds are always dangerous, and especially in wet seasons. When a sheep is infected with the rot, the white of the eyes looks dull, and they have a faint aspect; the animal is feeble, and his skin foul; the wool comes off in handsful at the least touch, and the gums look pale, and the teeth foul; he will also be dull and listless in motion, and heavy, as if his legs were not able to carry him. Many are generally affected at a time, and the first care must be to remove them from the sound ones, and put them in a close fold. They must have but little water, and their food must be hay and oats. Bleeding is destructive in the rot. The fact that sheep fed in salt marshes never have the rot, suggested salt as a remedy. It is a good preventive, and a cure. Though the farmer cannot rely with absolute certainty upon it, yet, among other remedies, it is highly useful. The following remedies and treatment have often effected cures:—

Bruise an ounce of the grains of paradise, and four ounces of juniper-berries, dried; add to these four pounds of bay salt, and half a pound of loaf-sugar; grind them well together, and sprinkle some of this upon the hay and oats that are given the sheep. Let this be continued three days, and look, from time to time, to the eyes, and examine every other way to see whether they mend or grow worse. If there be signs of amendment, let the same course be continued: if not, the following must be used:—Steep four pounds of antimony in two gallons of ale, for a week; then give the sheep this every night and morning, a quarter of a pint at a time. Boil a pound of the roots of avens, and two pounds of the roots of masterwort, in two gallons of water, till there are not more than six quarts remaining; strain this off, and press it hard; then pour a pint of it into a pailful of water that is to be given to the sheep for their drink. By these means, carefully managed, and under a good regulation in cleanness, dryness, and warmth, the rot will often be cured. This is all that can be promised; for there are times when the disease is so rooted, and when the temperature of the air so favors it, that nothing will get the better of it. If the sheep have a distaste to the food, because of the salt and other ingredients mixed among it, they must be omitted for two or three feedings, and then given in less quantity.

STRETCHES.—This is the name given to a disease which has been noticed among sheep. The name is exactly indicative of its effect on the animal; producing dislike to food, uneasiness, and a continual inclination to extend the fore and hind feet as far as possible, in the same manner the operation of stretching is performed by a horse or dog. The true remedy or rather preventive, would undoubtedly be a supply of green food; but we have never found anything more necessary, than a plentiful supply of salt, to remove the disease at once. In addition to this, we would recommend a spoonful of castor-oil to be given the sheep, repeating the dose, at suitable intervals, till the disease is removed.

TAR FOR SHEEP.

A gentleman who has a large flock of sheep says, that during the season of grazing he gives his sheep tar, at the rate of a gill a day to every twenty sheep. He puts the tar in troughs, sprinkles a little fine salt over it, and the sheep consume it with eagerness. This preserves them from worms in the head, promotes their health in general, and is thought to be a good specific against the rot.

DISEASE OF HOGS.

Hogs are subject to various diseases; but, according to Laurence, they are not easily doctored. They are subject to pox or measles, blood-striking, staggers, quinsy, indigestion, catarrh, peripneumonia, and inflammation of the lungs, called heavings. When not very sick, pigs will eat, and they will take medicine in their wash. When they will not, there is no help for them. As aperients, cleansers, and alteratives, sulphur, antimony, and madder, are our grand specifics, and are truly useful; as cordials and tonics, treacle and strong beer, in warm wash, and good peas and pollard; in the measles, sulphur, &c.; and if the patient require it, give cordials now and then in staggers, bleeding, fresh air, and perhaps niter; in catarrh a warm bed and warm cordial wash, and the same in quinsy or inflammation of the glands of the throat. If external suppuration appear likely, discharge the matter when ripe, and dress with tar and brandy, or balsam. The heavings, or unsoundness of the lungs in pigs, like the unsoundness of the liver in lambs, is sometimes found to be hereditary. There is no remedy. The disease in pigs is often in consequence of colds from wet lodgings, or hasty feeding in a poor state. In a certain stage it is highly inflammatory, and without remedy. Unction with train-oil, and the internal use of it, have been sometimes thought beneficial.

CURE FOR HOG CHOLERA.

The following remedy is confidently recommended, it having been used lately with decided success: —

One or two pounds of fresh tar; one pound of copperas, pulverized; half a pound of saltpeter, pulverized; six or eight pounds of ashes. Mix the above thoroughly, put in a trough, and add water. Should the hogs refuse to drink the mixture, add shelled corn, when they will eat it. The above quantity will be a dose for twenty-five or thirty head of hogs. Let the pigs have theirs in a trough to themselves. We advise fire-coals being kept on the ground where the hogs are fed.

TO CURE SWELLING OF THE THROAT IN HOGS.

Take of molasses one half-pint, and a tablespoonful of hog's lard melted; to this add one tablespoonful flour of sulphur; mix well, and drench the hog with it, and nine times out of ten it will be found to have the desired effect.

TO DESTROY VERMIN IN HOGS.

Mix a little tar with grease of any kind sufficient to make the tar thin; then, when fed sufficiently, pour it over the hogs, so as to have them well smeared with the tar. This may be repeated often in the summer and fall, or in good weather. You may give each hog a small tablespoonful of sulphur in their food, or in damp weather have them well sprinkled with strong wood-ashes; either of these remedies will prevent or destroy the vermin.

ANOTHER REMEDY.

Cut a few pods of red pepper in small pieces, and fry them in lard until they change their color; then mix it with tar and a small quantity of spirits of turpentine, and rub or smear it on the affected parts, and along the back and sides. It will effectually drive away the lice.

TO DESTROY WORMS IN THE KIDNEY OF HOGS.

Feed the hog with corn, boiled soft in strong ley, with the addition of a handful of charcoal. This feed is to be continued four or five days, by which time the hog will probably become as well as ever, and so continue thereafter.

CURE FOR THE MANGE IN HOGS.

Give them sulphur in their food, and wash them in soap-suds.

CURE FOR THE MANGE AND QUINSY IN HOGS.

The remedy for the mange is simply this: — Take the common poke-root, stalks and leaves, and boil a quantity of it until the liquid becomes quite strong; then season with salt, meal, pot-liquor, &c., until it is made palatable to the hog, and he will partake of it and the salad most bountifully. It has been observed, too, that if the hog has ticks on him, they all drop off after the first or second feed; but whether from the liquor getting on him, whilst feeding, or taking it inwardly, is not known. For the quinsy, give the hog tea, made strong, of pennyroyal, and seasoned as the poke-juice, with salt, meal, and pot-liquor. It may be repeated for two or three days till relief is given. Poke-root is a valuable medicine for many diseases incident to domestic animals. We believe a strong tea of poke-root, given frequently, will cure the malignant disease denominated Farcy. It acts upon the skin and the absorbents, and "cleanses the blood."

CURE OF MANGE IN DOGS.

Dipping the animal in a tan-vat several times a day for a week or so, has been known to make a complete cure.

ANOTHER REMEDY.

Mix pounded sulphur with common lard, and let the dog eat as much as he pleases; then anoint him well down the middle of his back, and behind his ears, with the balance. If repeated two or three times, this will certainly effect a cure.

BRIEF HINTS FOR WINTER.

Cattle, and all domestic animals, should commence the winter in good condition. Do not undertake to winter more cattle than you have means of providing for. Let every farmer aim to have the next spring, instead of thin, bony, slab-sided, shaggy cattle, fine, smooth, round, and healthy ones: and to this end, 1st. Let the cattle be well fed. 2d. Let them be fed regularly. 3d. Let them be properly sheltered from the pelting storm. Proper food, and regularity in feeding, will save flesh on the animal's back, and shelter will save the fodder. All domestic animals, in considerable numbers, should be divided into parcels and separated from each other, in order that the weaker may not suffer from the domination of the stronger, nor the diseased from the vigorous.

Farmers who have raised root-crops (and all good farmers have doubtless done so), should cut them up, and mix them with drier food, as meal, chopped hay, straw, or corn-stalks, and feed them to cattle or sheep.

Cow-houses and cattle-stables should be kept very clean, and well littered. To allow animals to lie down in the filth, which is sometimes suffered to collect in the stables, is exceedingly injurious and unwise.

By using beds of straw, or litter, the consequent quantity of manure will much more than repay the supposed waste of straw.

All stables should be properly ventilated.

Mixing food is generally better than feeding cattle on one substance alone. Cattle will generally eat straw with as much readiness as hay, if it is salted copiously, which may be done by sprinkling brine over it. A great saving is made by cutting small not only straw and corn-stalks, but hay also.

Sheep, as well as all other domestic animals, should have a constant supply of good water during the winter. They should also be properly sheltered from the inclement weather. In making them comfortable is to be found the great secret of keeping them in good condition. The farmer who disregards the comfort of domestic animals must not think it strange that his do not thrive and look as well as those of his neighbor, who may not allow them to suffer in this respect.

MISCELLANEOUS RECEIPTS.

METHOD OF REARING TURKEYS.

THE following curious method of rearing turkeys to advantage, is taken from a Swedish author: —

"Many of our housewives," he says, "have long despaired of success in rearing turkeys, and complain that the profit rarely indemnifies them for their trouble and loss of time, whereas little more is to be done than to plunge the chick into a vessel of cold water the very hour, if possible, but at least the very day that it is hatched, forcing it to swallow at least one whole peppercorn; after which let it be returned to its mother. From that time it will become hardy, and fear the cold no more than a hen's chicken. But it must be remembered that this useful species of fowls are also subject to one particular disorder when they are young, which often carries them off in a few days. When they begin to droop, examine carefully the feathers on the rump, and you will find two or three whose quill parts are filled with blood; upon drawing them the chick recovers, and after that requires no other care than what is commonly bestowed upon poultry that range the court-yard." The truthfulness of these assertions is well known in Sweden, where the plan has been highly successful for many years.

ANOTHER METHOD.

The principal remedy necessary, in the first instance, appears to be a stimulant, to counteract the extreme feebleness which attends young turkeys, more than other fowls, in the earliest stages of their existence; hence a grain of pepper, &c., is usually administered as soon as hatched. But instinct, their infallible guide, it appears, has more successfully directed them to the wild onion, which is proved to be a powerful restorative to their natures, and, in fact, a grand panacea to the race; when they are permitted to ramble, you will see them busily cropping the green blades of the onion with much apparent enjoyment. Small hominy made wet, with the addition of a portion of the wild onion chopped fine, or any other onion-tops that can be procured, affords the best and most wholesome food they can have, for several weeks at least, or so long as they are confined to small enclosures. Turkeys are very fond of green food of any kind, particularly lettuce and cabbage, the leaves of which may be chopped fine, and given them twice a day, morning and evening, with good effect. Continue also to feed them on hominy, so long as they may require your care, and the housewife, without uncommon accidents, will have no reason to complain of the loss of her turkeys.

ANOTHER METHOD.

When chickens are hatched out, let the hen and chickens be confined in a garden, or any other place where the young ones can sun themselves. Let them be fed with hominy for two or three days; then carry them to a rail pen, in a rye, oats, or buckwheat patch;

confine the hen, and feed at least three times a day with hominy, or small grain. The young ones will soon run about, catching insects, and will come to the hen's call. The hen should be thus confined until the turkeys are about half-grown; they will range about, but never out of the sound of the mother's call. The young ones are not so liable to injury from hawks or vermin, as when they follow the hen, in her rambles over the plantation; nor are they compelled, in keeping up with the hen, to fatigue themselves more than is good for health.

Great care must be taken to keep the pen dry; the foundation should be made higher, with dry sand, so as to admit of no standing water, and the top should be well covered to keep out the rain.

EGGS AND POULTRY.

Nearly every family can, with very little trouble, have eggs in plenty during the whole year, by putting in practice the following instructions: —

In the month of November, put apart eleven hens and a rooster, giving them a small chamber in the wood-house, defended from storms, and with an opening to the south. Place their food, water, and lime, on shelves convenient for them, with warm nests, and plenty of chalk nest-eggs. Those hens will lay, through the winter, on an average, six eggs daily. Whenever any of them are disposed to sit, that is, as soon as she begins to cluck, separate her from the others by a grated partition, and darken her apartment. These cluckers should be well attended and fed, and allowed to see, and partly associate, through the grates, with the other fowls; and as soon as the prisoner begins to sing, she should be liberated, and will very soon lay eggs. Egg-shells contain lime; therefore, when the earth is bound with frost, or covered with snow, if lime is not provided for chickens, they will not lay, or, if they do, the eggs must of necessity be without shells. Rubbish lime, from old chimneys and buildings, is proper, and only needs to be broken for them. They will often attempt to swallow pieces of lime-plaster as large as walnuts.

A dozen fowls shut up, away from the means of obtaining food, will require something more than a quart of Indian-corn a day; but, more or less, let them always have enough by them; and after they have become habituated to find enough at all times, a plenty in their little manger, they take but a few kernels at a time, except just before retiring to roost, when they will take nearly a spoonful into their crops; but if their provision comes to them scanted, or irregularly, they will take up a whole cropful at a time, and will stop laying.

A single dozen fowls, properly attended, will furnish a family with more than two thousand eggs in a year, and one hundred full-grown chickens for fall and winter stores. The expense of feeding the dozen fowls will not amount to eighteen bushels of Indian-corn. They may be kept in cities as well as in the country, and will do as well shut up the year round as to run at large; and a grated room, well lighted, ten feet by five, partitioned from any stable, or other out-house, is sufficient for the dozen fowls, with their roosting-places, nests, and feeding-troughs.

At the proper season, viz., in the spring of the year, five or six hens will hatch at the same time, and fifty or sixty chickens should be given to one hen.

Two hens will take care of one hundred chickens well enough, until they begin to climb their little stick roosts. They should then be separated from the hens entirely. They will wander less, and do better away from the fowls.

TO FATTEN FOWLS OR CHICKENS IN FOUR OR FIVE DAYS.

Set rice over the fire, with skimmed milk, only as much as will serve one day. Let it boil till the rice is quite swelled out, and feed the fowls three times a day with it. When you boil fresh rice, let the pans be set in water, that no sourness may be conveyed to the fowls, as that prevents them from fattening. Give them clean water to drink. By this method the flesh will have a clear whiteness, which no other food gives; and when it is considered how far a pound of rice will go, and how much time is saved by this mode, it will be found to be cheap.

TO CURE THE GAPES IN CHICKENS.

On the subject of this disease of chickens, a writer remarks: —

"On the dissection of chickens dying of this disease, it will be found that the windpipe contains numerous small worms, about half an inch in length, and the size of a small cambric needle. On the first glance, they would likely be mistaken for blood-vessels. These worms may be dislodged, and the disease cured, by the introduction of tobacco-smoke into the mouth, until the chicken becomes insensible. In this state it will remain for one or two minutes. The operation may be repeated, without endangering life.

34

The first application will usually produce the death or expulsion of the worms, and the removal of the affection; the second, always."

TO PREVENT DOGS FROM SUCKING EGGS.

Take of tartar emetic from four to eight grains, according to the age and strength of your dog; break the end of an egg, put in the tartar, and mix it. If your dog is disposed to suck eggs, he will readily eat it. Confine him from cold water. The next day repeat the dose, which continue to do on each succeeding day, until he refuses it, which will probably be the third or fourth day. After this, they will never be guilty of the like offence.

CAPONS.

Take the rooster (which should be about half-grown, or nearly so), lay him on the left side with the legs and wings extended; let your assistant hold him in that position; then, after picking away some of the feathers from the right side, with a sharp penknife, make an incision parallel with the ribs, just below them, about an inch and a half in length, taking care not to injure the intestines; then insert the thumb and fore-finger, and you will feel the testicles attached to the back-bone, not more than an inch from the incision, which you can remove with the thumb and finger with care; then sew up the incision in three or four stitches, and rub the wound with a little tar or grease. The fowls should be kept for a few days in a coop, and fed sparingly, after which they can be turned loose.

PRESERVATION OF EGGS, NO. I.

Relative to the preservation of eggs by immersion in lime-water, Mr. Peschier has given most satisfactory evidence of the efficacy of the process. Eggs, which he had preserved for six years in this way, being boiled and tried, were found perfectly fresh and good; and a confectioner of Geneva has used a whole cask preserved by the same means. In a small way eggs may be thus preserved in jars, or other vessels. They are to be introduced when quite fresh, the jar filled, after the eggs are put in, with lime-water, a little powdered lime sprinkled in at last, and then the jar closely corked. To prepare the lime-water, twenty or thirty pints of water are to be mixed up with five or six pounds of slacked quicklime put into a covered vessel, allowed to clear by standing, and the lime-water immediately used.

PRESERVATION OF EGGS, NO. II.

Eggs may, with proper care, be kept perfectly fresh, not only through the winter, but almost any length of time. The care necessary for this purpose is to render the shell impervious to the air; or to place them in such a situation that the yolk may not come directly in contact with the shell, but remain surrounded by the albumen or white, which is known to withstand the effects of the air much longer, without alteration, than the yolk. The eggs should be placed in a keg, on the small end; and every layer should be filled in with salt or sand, to keep them in that position. If they are wanted to be kept for any length of time, there should be a good coat on the top, and the keg headed up. It would be a great improvement to immerse the eggs previous to their being packed, in a mixture of lard or tallow and beeswax, with an addition of a small quantity of resin, to render the mixture more adhesive. Eggs thus prepared and packed, would continue good for a year or more.

PRESERVATION OF EGGS, NO. III.

One bushel of quicklime, thirty-two ounces of salt, eight ounces of cream of tartar. Mix the whole together, with as much water as will reduce the composition to such a consistency that an egg, when put into it, will swim. Then pack the eggs into jars, or kegs, and pour on the liquid till they are covered.

PRESERVING MILK.

A foreign journal states, that some milk was lately exhibited in Liverpool from on board a Swedish vessel, that was several months old, having made two voyages from Sweden to the West Indies and back again, and remained perfectly sweet and fresh. The manner of preparing it is as follows:—

The bottles are made clean and sweet, and the milk is milked directly into them, without the intervention of a pail. As fast as they are filled, they are closely corked, and the corks wired down as in bottling cider. The bottles are placed, when filled, in a boiler, a layer of straw, and a layer of bottles, until the layer is full. Fill the boiler with cold water, kindle a fire, and let it heat gradually; when it begins to boil, withdraw the fire, and let the bottles remain till cold. They must then be taken out, packed in hampers, with straw or sawdust, and stowed in the coolest part of the ship. The milk so exhibited was above eighteen months old, and was of excellent quality. It is evident this discovery will be the most available at sea; but where bottles could be easily obtained, many families living in cities and villages who keep a cow, might, by preserving some in this way, furnish themselves with a supply for the time a cow usually goes dry during the winter. In any event, the experiment could cost but little.

SUBSTITUTE FOR CREAM.

Beat up the whole of a fresh egg in a basin, and then pour boiling tea or water over it gradually, to prevent it curdling. In flavor and richness this preparation resembles cream.

PLAN OF AN ICE-HOUSE AND DAIRY.

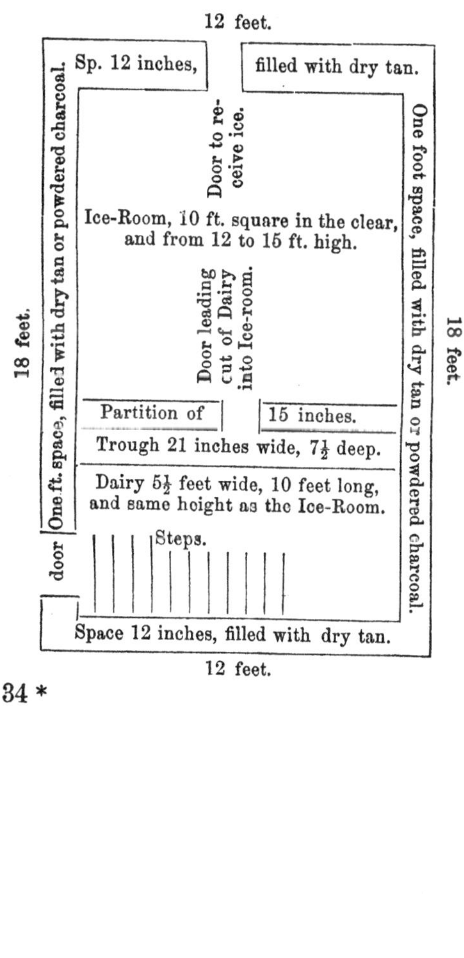

The above is the plan of an ice-house and dairy. The whole length eighteen feet, width twelve feet; the pit sunk six feet in the ground, and to the square above the common surface nine or ten feet. The house to be framed and finished in the common way, and weather-boarded. Another frame is made about two feet less every way, and put up inside of the frame just mentioned, the sills of which rest on the bottom of the pit, ceiled inside, with sleepers in the common way, and the space underneath and between the sleepers filled in with dry tan; floored with two-inch plank jointed, and the edges grooved and joints broken, so as to convey the water which drips from the ice into the dairy and trough. The partition which separates the dairy from the ice-room is double, and ceiled on both sides the space, which is about twelve to fifteen inches, and is filled with charcoal or dry tan. The ice-room and dairy are intended to be surrounded by dry tan or pulverized charcoal, which, as put in, ought to be rammed. The doors are all double, I mean one inside and one outside, both opening the same way; except the door of entrance into the dairy, the outside one opening to the outside, and the inside opening inside, as usual. The end door to receive the ice is four feet and a half high, and two feet nine inches wide, and the space between the two doors, about a foot, after the ice-room is filled, is packed full of straw. The facings of the doors between the dairy and ice-room are covered with thick woollen selvage, fastened on with small tacks, so as to prevent, as far as possible, the access of warm air. Into one of these doors there are driven several hooks, such as butchers use, on which to hang fresh meat; and the temperature in that open space being 40°, it can be kept there sound and fresh as long as desired. The temperature of the dairy is 49°; the dairy has several shelves, on which to place meats, butter, jars of preserves, &c. &c.; the milk in pans is put in the trough which receives the drippings from the ice. The flight of steps must be narrow, and have a railing as a safeguard. Embankments of clay are made all around the house, to rise perhaps two or three feet above the common surface, so as to carry off the water as it may fall.

The above is better than a spring-house or dairy, and answers the purpose of both. In taking out the ice, enter the doors leading out of the dairy into the ice-room, beginning, of course, at the bottom of the ice instead of the top, as usual; the ice-room holds about one thousand bushels. The charcoal, when used, ought to be pounded small, or if passed through a bark-mill would perhaps be better; it ought to be fresh. If tan be used, it must be dry; and either, when put in, ought to be rammed. The space between the frames above the ground ought to be from two to four feet. Care must be taken in constructing the frame, especially the inside one, to give it sufficient height to allow the door of entrance into the dairy to be about six feet.

The dairy is without a floor. The floor of the ice-room must be somewhat lower where it enters the dairy than at the other end, and the plank forming the floor of the ice-room must project into the dairy over the sleeper a few inches, so that the water running from the floor may fall into the trough, which is made water-tight. No straw is used about the ice. The ice-room is floored above, and covered with charcoal and tan to the thickness of two to four feet.

A PORTABLE ICE-HOUSE.

Take an iron-bound butt or puncheon, and knock out the head, cutting a very small hole in the bottom, about the size of a wine-cork; place inside of it a wooden tub, shaped like a churn, resting it upon two pieces of wood, which are to raise it from touching the bottom. Fill the space round the inner tub with pounded charcoal, and fit to the tub a cover, with a convenient handle, having inside one or two small hooks, on which are to be hung the bottles during the operation; place on the lid a bag of charcoal, about two feet square; if the charcoal in this bag is pounded, it will answer better; and over all place another cover, which must cover the head of the outer cask. When the apparatus is thus prepared, let it be placed in a cold cellar, and buried in the earth about four-fifths of its length; but though cold, the cellar must be dry; wet ground will not answer, and a sandy soil is the best. Fill the inner tub, or nearly so, with pounded ice; or if prepared in the winter, with snow well pressed down, and the apparatus will be complete. Whenever it is wished to make ice, take off the upper cover, then the sack or bag of pounded charcoal, and suspend the vessel containing the water or liquid to be frozen to the hooks inside of the inner cover; then close up the whole, as before, for half an hour, taking proper care to exclude the external air.

PLAN OF A KENTUCKY BEE-HOUSE.

The building to be twelve feet long, eight wide, and seven high from the floor to the plate or ceiling (the floor being eighteen inches from the ground), and is to consist of four posts, weather-boarded round, and covered in, to prevent the bees from getting in the house; they being confined in six boxes, three on either side of the house, placed fifteen inches one above another. This drawing (fig. 24) represents one side of the house, viewed from the outside.

Fig. 24.

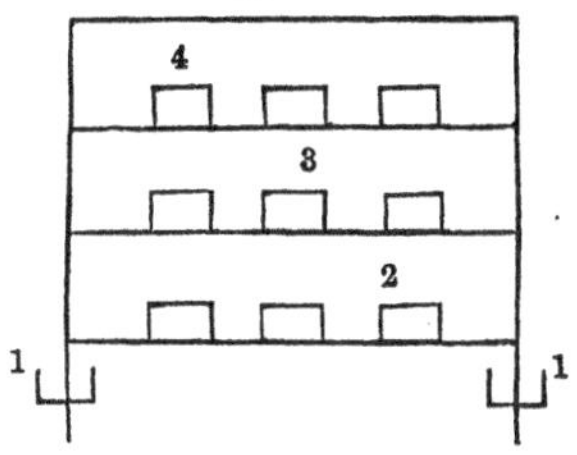

Fig. 25.

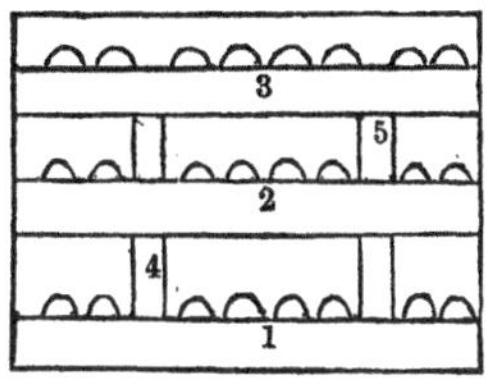

Fig. 24. Nos. 1, 1, are copper troughs running round the post, half-way between the floor and ground, which are kept filled with water to prevent ants or other insects from getting in the house. Nos. 2, 3, and 4, are tubes eight inches wide, and one-quarter of an inch deep, to convey the bees through the wall into the long boxes, and entering them at the bottom, there being three to each long box. The drawing, fig. 25, represents one side of the house, viewed from the inside. Nos. 1, 2, and 3, are long boxes, eighteen inches wide, and twelve deep, extending the whole length of the house, with eight holes, four inches square, in each box, upon which are set caps of two gallons, with two half-inch holes in each, one near the top, the other about the center of the cap, in which the smoke of a burning rag is blown to drive the bees from the cap into the long box. A knife or wire should be drawn under the cap, to separate the comb from the box, when the cap of

honey may be removed, and an empty one put in its place. Nos. 4 and 5, are tubes, three inches square, to convey the bees from one box to another, that one swarm may do the whole; or if one or more swarms be put in each box, that they may become as one, as they will not have more than one queen when put together, by which they are prevented from destroying themselves by fighting. A house of this description, when the long boxes are filled, will afford, at a moderate calculation, ninety-six gallons of honey, in the comb, annually.

ANOTHER PLAN.

Several individuals have tried this arrangement with entire success. It consists of a house of brick or wood (of wood standing on blocks, or it might be made with good solid posts set in the ground), say of the size of a common smoke-house, with a door to admit of the entrance of a man. The inside is merely furnished with shelves like an ordinary pantry. The bees pass in and out through several apertures resembling spouts, arranged in rows on each side. These spouts project six inches, and the hole is perhaps two or three inches wide, by from one-eighth to one-half an inch in height. The benefits of this method are said to be these:—The bees never swarm, but continue filling up the house. The honey may be easily taken out when the bees retire to the bottom of the combs in cold weather, and it is said to be an infallible preventive of worms.

TAKING HIVES WITHOUT DESTROYING THE BEES.

Having always thought that there was inhumanity in the old plan of destroying the bees in order to take the honey, we determined to try the more humane plan practised by the French of robbing them of their sweets without depriving them of life, and we have put the plan twice into operation the present season with entire success. The method, which is easy, is as follows: — In the dusk of the evening, when the bees are quietly lodged, place a tub near the hive; then throw the hive over with its bottom upward into the tub; cover the hive with a clean one, which must be previously prepared by washing its inside with salt and water, and rubbing it with hickory leaves, thyme, or some other aromatic leaves or herbs. Having carefully adjusted the mouth of each hive to the other, so that no aperture remains between them, take a small stick and gently beat around the sides of the full hive for about fifteen minutes, in which time the bees will leave their cells in the lower hive, and ascend and adhere to the upper one. Then gently lift the new hive, with all its little tenants, and place it on the stand from which the other hive was taken. This should be done about midsummer, so as to allow the bees time to provide a new stock of honey for winter's use.

HUNTING BEES.

The manner of hunting bees, as practised in the new settlements, may be familiar to many, but perhaps not to all. As advantage is taken of a peculiar instinct, it would, probably, be interesting to those unacquainted with it, to be informed of the process. A tin box is provided, capable of containing about a pint. Into this is put a piece of dry honey-comb; a bottle of honey and water mixed, about half and half, is also provided. The honey is diluted, in order that it may be more readily poured into the dry comb, that the bees may not be so liable to get it upon their wings, and will be able to fill themselves more expeditiously. Apparatus for making a fire may also be necessary. With these the hunter proceeds to a newly-cleared field, at a distance from any hive of domestic bees; and having poured a little of the composition into the comb, he proceeds to search among the wild flowers for a bee. If one can be found, he is caught in the box by shutting the lid over him. As soon as he becomes still, the lid is carefully removed, when he will be found busily filling himself with honey. When he rises he must be watched in order to ascertain his course. After making one or two circuits about the box, he will fly off in a straight course to his home. After an absence of a few minutes, say five or ten, he will return, bringing with him two or three of his companions. These will soon fill themselves, go home, and return again with a number more. Thus they will continue to increase in number till, in the course of half an hour, there will be one hundred or more in the box. By that time the line will be ascertained with precision. The lid is now shut over as many as possible, and the box is removed on the line to the edge of the woods, where it is again opened. The line will soon be found at the new station, as before, and thus the box is removed from station to station, until the whole tree is either discovered or passed. If the tree be passed, the line, of course, will be retrograde. A small pocket spyglass is a convenient thing for searching the tops of trees, as it requires a good eye to see a bee at that distance. If a bee cannot be found to commence operations with, a little honey is burned on a stone; and if a wandering bee happens to be near, he will be attracted by the smell. The proper time for hunting bees is on a fair warm day in the month of September or October. During the summer months, when food for bees is to be found everywhere, they will not traverse. If a bee tree is in the neighborhood of a sugar camp, bees will be found about the tree in the time of making sugar.

FISH PONDS.

Perhaps it is not generally known that many kinds of fish at present found in salt water may be taken thence to fresh water, and that they will not deteriorate in flavor. They may thus be transplanted into our fresh water ponds, where they will speedily multiply, and become, not only gratifying to the palate, but actually a source of profit. Experiments have been made in Europe, and in this country, and the fact is there rendered beyond dispute, that flounders, bass, cod, mackerel, and eels (and to this list may be added crabs, oysters, mussels, shrimps), all live and do well in fresh water. Many of them, when thus transferred, improve in size and delicacy.

PRESERVATION OF APPLES.

Apples, after remaining as long on the trees as safety from the frost will permit, should be picked carefully by hand, put into close casks, and kept dry and cool as possible. If suffered to lie on the floor for weeks, they will wither and lose their flavor, without acquiring any additional durability. The best mode of preparing apples for spring use is the putting of them in dry sand as soon as picked. For this purpose, dry the sand in the heat of summer; and, late in October, put down the apples in layers singly, with a covering of sand upon each layer. The singular advantages of this mode of treatment are these: first, the sand keeps the apples from the air, which is essential to their preservation; secondly, the sand checks the evaporation of the apples, thus preserving them in their full flavor, at the same time any moisture yielded by the apples (and some there will be) is absorbed by the sand, so that the apples are kept dry, and all mustiness is prevented. The casks should be headed.

Irish potatoes will keep in a good state put up in the same way, but should be dried a few days in the shade after digging, spreading them thinly on the ground or floor.

TO PRESERVE GRAPES AND PLUMS IN A FRESH STATE.

Grapes or plums may be preserved in a fresh state for use, for a length of time, by alternating them in layers with cotton battings, in a large stone jar, and placing them in a chamber secure from frost.

TO KEEP PLUMS AND PEACHES FRESH THROUGH THE YEAR.

Beat well up together equal quantities of honey and spring water; put it into an earthen vessel; put in the fruits, all freshly gathered, and cover them quite close. When any of the fruit is taken out, wash it in cold water, and it is fit for immediate use.

TO PRESERVE PUMPKINS IN A FRESH STATE.

Pull them after they have their growth, and a little before the frost comes on, and put them in a warm, dry room. By this method they have been kept in a dry state for two years.

TO PRESERVE GREEN CORN FOR BOILING.

Pluck the corn when fit for eating; strip down the husk so as to remove the silk, and then replace it. Pack it away in a barrel, and pour on strong pickle, such as is used for meat, with a weight to keep it down. When boiled, it will be perfectly fresh and sweet as when taken from the stock.

PRESERVATION OF CABBAGES.

After they have their growth, and are gathered in the fall, cut off their loose leaves and stalks, that nothing may remain but the sound part of the head, and put them up in a tight cask. By thus excluding them from the air, they may be kept for a long time.

TO PRESERVE GREEN PEAS.

Gather them while they are yet tender; shell and dry them. If they can be dried in the shade without molding, so much the better. The following winter, after soaking them in warm water over-night, you will find them swollen to the same size, and being as green and tender as they were when gathered. Then boil them as usual, and you will have green peas in midwinter.

TO PRESERVE TOMATOES IN A FRESH STATE.

Tomatoes may be kept fresh through the fall and winter, by packing them in jars, laying alternately a layer of dry sand a layer of tomatoes, until the vessel is full; after which, cover them up tight to keep the air out, and place them in a dry cellar.

TO DRY CHERRIES.

To every five pounds of cherries, stoned, weigh one of sugar double-refined; put the fruit into a preserving-kettle, with very little water; make both scalding hot; take the fruit, and immediately dry them; put them into a kettle again, stirring the sugar between each layer of cherries. Let it stand to melt; then set the kettle on the fire, and make it scalding hot as before; take it off, and repeat this thrice with the sugar; drain them from the syrup, and lay them singly to dry on dishes in the sun, or on the stove. When dry, put them into a sieve, dip it into a pan of cold water, and draw it instantly out again, and pour them on a fine, soft cloth; dry them, and set them once more in the hot sun, or on a stove; keep them in a box, with layers of white paper, in a dry place. This way is the best to give plumpness to the fruit, as well as color and flavor.

DRIED APPLES AND PEARS.

In France, apples and pears are prepared in the following manner: —

The fruit, with the stems left on, to prevent any loss of juice, is put into boiling water, in which it is left until it becomes soft. It is then taken out and carefully peeled, and placed on a strainer, under which is a dish to catch the juice; when peeled, it is put into an oven heated to the ordinary temperature for bread, and left there twenty-four hours. When taked out, and cold, the fruit is pressed flat, and after being plunged into its own juice, which has been set apart for that purpose, it is packed in boxes and exported. For family use, it might be packed away in stone jars.

DRIED PEACHES.

Just before fully ripe, peel peaches, take out the nuts, put them in boiling water till they are a little soft; take them out, and throw them into a pailful of cold water; when cold, drain and weigh them. To every pound of peaches put half a pound of powdered loaf-sugar. Lay the peaches in a kettle, and sprinkle the sugar until it is all in. Let it remain until the syrup runs sufficiently to allow putting it on over a very slow fire. Let them boil slowly till the peaches look clear; then put them in a large bowl, and let them remain all night. The next morning place them snugly in dishes, and put them into the sun to dry. Turn them over every day until they are sufficiently dry to be packed in boxes or jars.

VINEGAR.

Put a gallon of good vinegar in a tight cask, and place it in a cellar, occasionally shaking it around, for a day or two. Then commence filling up the cask gradually with whiskey and water, in the proportion of one gallon of the former to eight of the latter. It is best not to fill up too fast at first, but wait a week or two before adding again. By this process, an abundant supply of the purest vinegar may always be kept on hand.

STARCH.

In making starch from wheat, the grain is steeped in cold water until it becomes soft, and yields a milky juice by pressure; it is then put into sacks of linen, and pressed in a vat, filled with cold water, as long as any milky juice exudes. After standing some time, the fluid gradually becomes clear, and a white powder, which is starch, remains at the bottom.

ATTAR OF ROSES.

The following is an account of the manner in which this costly perfume is prepared in the East: —

Steep a large quantity of the petals of roses, freed from every extraneous matter, in pure water, in an earthen or wooden vessel, which is exposed daily to the sun, and housed at night, till a scum rises to the surface. This is the attar, which is carefully absorbed by a very small piece of cotton tied to the end of a stick. The oil collected, squeeze out of the cotton into a vial; stop it for use. The collection of it should be continued whilst any scum is produced.

SODA FOR WASHING.

To five gallons of water add a pint and a half of soap, and two ounces subcarbonate of soda; put the clothes (after soaking over-night) into the mixture when at boiling heat, rubbing the parts most soiled with soap. Boil them one hour, drain, rub, and rinse them in warm water: after being put into indigo water, they are fit for drying. Half the soap, and more than half the labor, is saved by washing in this manner.

TO MAKE SOFT SOAP.

Take five bushels of ashes, damp them thoroughly on the ground, and let them stand from five hours to two days, as may be convenient. Then make up the heap in an oblong form, open the middle, and put in three pecks of perfectly fresh lime; sprinkle about three or four quarts of water over it, and cover up. Use hot water in very cold weather, or in large experiments cold water will answer in any weather. In half an hour the lime will heat and burst open the heap of ashes, when the whole must be well and quickly mixed, and put into the ley-tub to the depth of one foot, and beaten moderately; another layer of ashes, the same depth as the first, is then to be added and beaten as before, and so on until the tub is filled within six inches of the top; water is then to be poured in steadily until the ashes are nearly or entirely spent. The ley must be of a strength scarcely sufficient to float a newly-laid egg: four gallons of this ley are to be put into a large kettle, and thirty or forty pounds of fat or grease added, and well stirred over a gentle heat. When it is perceived that the sharp taste of the mixture is lost, more ley is to be added occasionally, until the soap becomes transparent and very thick, and toward the last of the operation, the liquid must be made to boil briskly. When the soap is made, let it stand for a day, and if it does not grow thin in that time, no apprehensions need be excited in that respect. The kettle should be covered, and should hold more liquid than it is intended to boil, to give room for a brisk ebullition toward the close.

TO MAKE HARD SOAP.

Mild ley is to be used. When the soft soap is finished, and the mixture still tolerably hot, add sea salt (or alum salt), until the ley drops clear from the soap. If it closes, add more salt, and at the same time slacken the fire; then boil until the froth becomes as light as a feather. Draw the fire, and pour salt and water into the mixture to cool it, observing to make a rapid stream, and not to let any drops fall in turning the bucket. When the soap is too strong of the alkali, it will not grain: in that case, add clean fat by degrees until it granulates, stirring it all the time over a gentle heat: when it boils, no more fat need be added. It is to be observed that if the ashes have been too tightly pressed in the ley-tub, the ley will not filtrate; and if they have not been sufficiently pressed, the water will run foul. In the first case, the ashes may be loosened with a long iron skewer; in the latter, they must remain some hours to settle, and also be pressed.

TO MAKE COLD SOAP.

The leach-tub, or hogshead, must be covered at the bottom with straw and sticks; then put in a bushel of ashes, then two or three quarts of unslacked lime, upon which you must throw two quarts of boiling water to excite fermentation and slack; put in another bushel of ashes, and as much more lime and water, and continue to do so until your vessel is full; put in hot water until you can draw off the ley, after which the heat of the water is not of much consequence. You must have at least two-thirds of a bushel of lime to a hogshead, if you wish your soap to be made quickly: one hogshead of ashes will make two barrels of soap. When you draw off your ley, you must keep the first two pailsful by themselves, and the next two in another vessel, and the third two in another vessel still; then weigh twenty-nine pounds of clear strained grease, or of scraps without straining, thirty pounds; put into a large kettle with three pounds of resin; then pour over it one pailful of ley from the first vessel, and one from the second vessel; put it over the fire, and let it boil twenty minutes: be careful to add no ley over the fire, but swing off the crane if it is in danger of boiling over; put it into your barrel, and put in one pailful of ley from the third vessel, and give it a good stir: then weigh your grease for another barrel, and take the ley remaining in the vessels in the same manner as for the first barrel; then draw off your weak ley, and fill up the vessels as fast as possible, remembering to put half in each barrel, that they may be equally strong: if the leach run through fast, you may have the barrels full in an hour, and so hard that you can hardly stir them. You must stir it after you put in the ley, till the barrel is full. Fourteen quarts of melted grease is the quantity for a barrel.

A SIMPLE METHOD OF MAKING SOAP.

To thirty-two gallons of ley, of strength just sufficient to bear an egg, add sixteen pounds of clean, melted grease, which, by being placed in the hot sun, and occasionally stirred, will, in a few days, produce a soap of the first quality.

MAKING DIPPED CANDLES.

The tallow, when melted, should be ladled into a wooden vessel of convenient width and depth, which has been previously heated by filling it with boiling water for an hour or more. Fill the vessel within an inch of the top with melted tallow, and keep it that height by adding hot tallow or hot water. By this means the candles will be kept of a full size at the top, and not taper off to a point, as is often seen with the country candles. The tallow, when used for dipping candles, should not be too hot. A temperature that will allow the finger to be dipped in without burning, is sufficiently hot, and at this temperature the tallow will take on the wicks very fast. The wicks should be lowered into the melted tallow very gradually, and should be lifted out of the tallow so slowly that when the buttons of the candles are clear from the surface of the melted tallow, no tallow will run off them. When the candles are raised quickly out of the melted tallow, the tallow will run off the candles in a stream; whereas if the candles are raised out slowly, not a particle of tallow will fall from the candles. A few trials will satisfy any person in this matter. If the tallow is boiling hot, the wick will not take the tallow to any considerable extent. When candles are raised out of the tallow rapidly, the candles will be large at the bottom, and the tallow will extend below the wick, so that when burnt in the candlestick, a piece of the candle will have no wick in it; and therefore, for burning, will be useless. Where people have no suitable wooden vessel, an iron vessel will answer for a dipping vessel. When tallow has been thoroughly melted over the fire, should it be dirty or impure, throw into it, while hot, a small quantity of finely-powdered alum, and in a short time a scum will be seen rising to the surface, in appearance like dirty froth. Skim this off as it rises. This scum will rise for half an hour or more.

Prepare your wicks about half the usual size, and wet them thoroughly with spirits of turpentine, put them in the sun until dry, and then mold or dip your candles. Candles thus made, last longer, and give a much clearer light. In fact they are nearly or quite equal to sperm, in clearness of light.

A NEW WAY TO MAKE CANDLES.

We have been shown a candle, about the size of a broom straw, which makes a very brilliant light, and is as durable as the tallow candle. As this is the age for economy in everything, it may not be amiss for us to tell our readers how to make them. Take one pound of beeswax, and a fourth of a pound of soft turpentine from the tree, melt them together; strain them; take your wick of the desired length, and stretch it as you would in making a plow line; then take the composition in a thin waiter, and hold the wick down in it as you apply it from end to end; this done three times will complete the operation. The above proportion of the ingredients is sufficient for a wick forty yards long.

TO DYE COTTON YARN A DEEP BLUE.

Take one pound of logwood, chipped fine, or pounded; boil it in a sufficient quantity of water, until all the substance is out of it; then take about half a gallon of the liquor, and dissolve in it half an ounce of alum, and one ounce of verdigris; boil your yarn in the logwood-water one hour, stirring and keeping it loose. Take out your yarn, mix the half-gallon that contains the verdigris and alum; then put your yarn into the mixture, and boil it four hours, stirring it and keeping it loose all the time, and taking it out once every hour to give it air; after which, dry it, then boil it in soap and water, and it is done. The above will dye six pounds of yarn an elegant deep blue; after which put in as much yarn into the same liquor, and boil it three hours, stirring it as before, and you will have a good pale blue; or boil hickory bark in your liquor, and you will have an elegant green.

TO COLOR GREEN.

Take half a pound of oil of vitrol, one ounce of indigo, pulverized; put them in a bottle, shake it repeatedly three or four days; then put it in a hickory bark dye, with two pounds of alum. This mixture will cover twelve pounds of yarn: it is to be simmered over the fire several hours, frequently taking it out to air on a pole, over the kettle: you can dye it in iron, copper, or brass. When the yarn is dry, wash it in cold water; the hickory dye is to be taken off the fire, when the mixture is put in out of the bottle, or it will run over; for the hickory dye must be boiling hot when it is put in.

TO COLOR RED.

To three pounds of yarn, take one pound of alum, and one pound of madder; dissolve the alum in a sufficient quantity of water to cover the yarn; scald it well in that water; then rinse it well in pure water; mix wheat bran and water to the consistence of thin gruel, a sufficient quantity to cover the yarn well; mix the madder well in this preparation; put in the yarn, and boil two or three hours, stirring and keeping it loose in the vessel. If you do not wish it deep, take it out in a very short time; but if you wish a deep color, let it remain several hours. Rinse it in cold water, after letting it air. The bran must be boiled the night before.

TO DYE RED, WITH REDWOOD.

One pound of redwood (chipped fine), two ounces of alum, powdered; the redwood must stand twenty-four hours in river or spring water; then boil it well, and after straining, mix your alum and aquafortis, and boil it well for several hours. Mix one ounce aquafortis, one ounce block tin, in a tumbler, and set it in the sun about one hour. The above will color two pounds of yarn. After being dried, wash out with soft soap.

TO DYE CRIMSON.

To two gallons of the juice of pokeberries, when they are quite ripe, add half a gallon of strong cider-vinegar, to dye one pound of wool, which must be first washed very clean with hard soap; the wool, when wrung dry, is to be put into the vinegar and pokeberry juice, and simmered in a copper vessel for one hour; then take it out, let it drip a while, and spread it in the sun. The vessel must be free from grease of any kind.

TO DYE PINK.

Two ounces cochineal, two pounds of cream tartar, one pound of alum, the whole put in a kettle of soft water; then put in six pounds of clean yarn, and boil it well; it is not to be washed after being dried.

TO COLOR YELLOW.

Take three-fourths of hickory bark, with the outside shaved off, and one-fourth of black-oak bark, done in the same manner; boil them well together in a bell-metal kettle, until the color is deep; then add alum sufficient to make it foam when stirred up; put your yarn in, and let it simmer a little while; then take it out and air it, repeating the process two or three times, and having a pole over the kettle to hang it on, so that it may drain in the kettle; when dry, rinse it in cold water.

COLORING FLANNEL.

Take black alder bark, boil it well, then skim or strain it well; wet the cloth in a pretty strong ley, and dip it into the alder liquor: let it remain till cool enough to wring, and you will have an indelible orange color. The better the cloth, the better the color.

NANKEEN COLOR.

A pailful of ley, with a piece of copperas half as big as a hen's egg boiled in it, will dye a fine nankeen color, which will never wash out.

METHOD OF CLEANSING SILK, WOOLLEN, AND COTTON GOODS, WITHOUT DAMAGE TO THE TEXTURE OR COLOR.

Take raw potatoes in the state they are taken out of the earth, wash them well; then rub them on a grater, over a vessel of clean water, to a fine pulp; pass the liquid matter through a coarse sieve into another tub of clean water. Let the mixture stand, till the fine white particles of the potatoes are precipitated; then pour off the mucilaginous liquor, and preserve it for use. The article to be cleansed should then be laid upon a linen cloth on a table, and having provided a clean sponge, dip it in the potato liquor, apply this sponge, thus wet, upon the article to be cleansed, and rub it well upon it with repeated portions of the potato liquor, till the dirt is perfectly separated; then wash the article in clear water several times, to remove the loose dirt. It may afterwards be smoothed or dried. Two middle-sized potatoes will be sufficient for a pint of water.

The coarse pulp which does not pass the sieve is of great use in cleansing worsted curtains, tapestry, carpets, or other coarse goods. It is also useful in cleansing oil-paintings, or furniture that is soiled. Dirty painted wainscots may be cleaned by wetting a sponge in the liquor, then dipping it in a little fine, clean sand, and afterwards rubbing the wainscot with it.

TO CLEAN SILK STOCKINGS.

Wash your stockings first with white soap and lukewarm water, to take out the rough dirt; then rinse them in fair water, and work them well in a fresh soap-water; make a third soap-water pretty strong and hot, in which put a little stone blue, wrapped in a flannel bag, till the water is blue enough; then wash your stockings well therein, and wring them. Let them be dried so that they may remain a little moist, then fumigate them with brimstone; after which put upon a wooden leg two stockings, one upon the other, observing that the two fronts, or outsides, are face to face; then polish them with a glass.

TO TAKE STAINS OUT OF SILK.

Mix together in a vial two ounces of essence of lemon, and one more of oil of turpentine. Grease and other spots in silk are to be rubbed gently with a fine rag, dipped in the above composition.

TO TAKE SPOTS OUT OF SILK OR LINEN.

Of spirits of turpentine, twelve drops, and the same quantity of spirits of wine; grind these with an ounce of pipe-makers' clay, and cover the spots therewith. You are to wet the composition when you do either silk, linen, or woollen with it. Let it remain till dry, then rub it off, and the stains or spots will disappear. True spirits of salt, diluted with water, will remove iron-molds from linen; and sal-ammoniac, with lime, will take out the stains of wine.

ANOTHER METHOD.

Magnesia, if you have not French chalk, will effectually remove grease-spots from silk, on rubbing it in well; and after standing a while, apply a piece of soft brown paper to the wrong side, on which press a warm iron gently; and what grease is not absorbed by the paper, can be removed by washing the spot carefully with cold water.

TO WASH SILK.

Lay the piece of silk upon a clean board; soap a piece of flannel well, without making it very wet, and with this rub the silk carefully and evenly one way. After having thus cleansed one side of the silk, take a wet sponge and wash the soap; proceed in the same manner to clean the other side, and then wipe the water off each with a clean, dry cloth; after which, hang it as singly as possible upon a linen horse, and let it dry gradually. When very nearly dry, iron it.

TO MAKE CALICO WASH WELL.

Infuse three gills of salt in four quarts of boiling water; put the calico in while it is hot, and leave it till cold. In this way the colors are rendered permanent, and will not fade by subsequent washing.

TO REMOVE IRON MOLDS FROM LINEN.

Hold the iron mold on the cover of a tankard of boiling water, and rub on the spots a little juice of sorrel and salt; when the cloth has thoroughly imbibed the juice, wash it in ley.

TO TAKE MILDEW OUT OF LINEN.

Take soap, and rub it well in the linen; then scrape some fine chalk, and rub that also in the linen. Lay it on the grass; as it dries, wet it a little, and it will come out at twice doing.

TO TAKE INK OR WINE OUT OF LINEN OR WOOLLEN.

Take the juice of lemons, or sorrel, and wet the spot with it several times, letting it dry each time; then wash it with soap and vinegar, and the spot will go out.

TO REMOVE INK SPOTS FROM LINEN.

Lemon-juice will effectually remove ink from linen or muslin, if applied before the article has been washed. But as persons in the country may not be able at all times to get a lemon, I would advise them to buy a small bottle of vitriol. A few drops of this acid, mixed with pure water, and applied to the spots of ink, will entirely remove them. Great caution must be observed, however, not to suffer any part of the linen, or other material, to come in contact with the acid before it is sufficiently diluted: otherwise, the texture of the fabric will be destroyed.

TO REMOVE FRUIT STAINS.

These are readily removed from clothes by wetting them, and placing them near lighted brimstone. A few matches will answer the purpose.

TO KEEP OFF MOTHS.

In the month of April, or before flies or insects make their appearance, beat your fur or woollen garments well with a small cane or elastic stick; then wrap them up in linen, observing not to press the fur garments too hard, and put between the folds some camphor in small lumps; then put your articles in boxes well closed. When the garments are wanted for use, take them out, beat them well as before, and expose them twenty-four hours to the air, which will take away the smell of the camphor.

TO BLEACH BEESWAX.

Melt your wax, and while hot throw it into cold water to reduce it into small pieces, or spread it out into very thin leaves, and lay it out in the sun and air for a few days on linen cloths; then melt it over again, and expose it as before, till the sun and dew have bleached it; then, for the last time, melt it in a kettle, and cast it with a ladle on a table covered over with little round, hollow molds in the form of the casks sold by the apothecaries; but first wet your molds with cold water, that the wax may be the easier got out; lastly, lay it out in the air for two or three days and nights, to make it more transparent and dry.

SIMPLE MEANS OF PURIFYING WATER.

It is not generally known, as it ought to be, that pounded alum possesses the property of purifying water. A large tablespoonful of pulverized alum, sprinkled into a hogshead of water (the water being fresh at the time), will, after the lapse of a few hours, by precipitating to the bottom the impure particles, purify it, so that it will be found to possess nearly all the freshness and clearness of the finest spring-water; a pailful, containing four gallons, may be purified with a single teaspoonful.

TO MAKE A MATTRASS, THAT WILL NOT SINK IN THE MIDDLE.

To produce this effect, make your mattrass twice as long as usual, double it, sew the two ends together, and arrange the stuffing, where it joins, the same as the rest. It will then have the form of a roller, or double towel, which may be rolled for ever, and will always remain double and folded. When you put it on the bed, it will be the same as two mattrasses one over the other. It takes no more tucking or stuffing for this double mattrass than for two single ones. The advantage of this invention is, that every time the bed is made, you may easily roll the mattrass, so that the part which was under the body may be placed at the head or foot, sometimes above and sometimes below; and successively every part of the mattrass made to pass to those places where the compression is greater: you may even, from time to time, turn it inside out like a stocking, and by this means produce other changes. A mattrass made in this manner lasts much longer, and is likewise easier to sleep on than one made in the usual way.

TO DESTROY RATS.

Take a few fresh corks, rasp them fine, and fry them in the common way with a little butter or fat; place it, while warm, at the points where rats are plenty, and, if possible, where they may eat the dose undisturbed by any noise; leave no water within their reach, and in a few days not a vestige of the creatures will be seen. The above plan is more safe than poisoning them.

ANOTHER METHOD.

Take a small pine stick, and slightly fasten six or eight fish-hooks to it, the points all one way, and put the stick in the rat-holes, so that when they run into the hole they will rub against the hooks, which will catch into the skin, and with a little exertion they clear the hooks from the stick, and go off squealing with the hooks fast in the skin; and a few rats, so hooked, will give warning to others, and they will all soon disappear. Try it, and you will not be disappointed.

TO PREVENT FLEAS INFESTING ROOMS OR BEDS.

Take a few branches of pennyroyal, and hang it up or lay it on the bed, or carry a few sprigs in the pocket, and the flea will never make its appearance. This simple remedy has never failed of the desired effect.

A CURE FOR THE RED ANTS.

Common salt is a complete barrier to the approach of the red ant. Let the salt be so placed, that they cannot approach the place from which you wish to exclude them, without passing over it, and the remedy is complete.

TO DESTROY FLIES.

Half a spoonful of ground black pepper, one teaspoonful of brown sugar, one tablespoonful of cream, mixed well together, and placed on a plate, will attract and destroy flies, without any danger of poisoning children.

A SIMPLE WAY OF PREVENTING FLIES FROM SITTING ON PICTURES, OR ANY OTHER FURNITURE.

Let a large bunch of leeks soak for five or six days in a pailful of water, and wash your pictures, or any piece of furniture, with it. The flies will never come near anything so washed.

TO DESTROY ROACHES.

Preserve a moderate quantity of pokeroot, boil it in water until the juice is extracted, and mingle the liquor with good molasses; spread the liquor in platters or soup-plates in the kitchen, pantry, closet, wash-house, or whatever apartment is infested by them, and the enemy will be found slain in heaps by the following morning.

TO CLEAN FLINT GLASS BOTTLES, DECANTERS, ETC.

Roll up, in small pieces, some white, brown, or blotting paper; then wet and soap the same; put them into the vessel to be cleaned, with a little warm water; shake them well for a few minutes, then rinse with clean water, and it will be as bright and clear as when new from the shops.

TO CLEAN SILVER AND PLATED WARE.

Wash it first in warm water, to take off grease, or any kind of dirt; then wipe it dry with a soft towel. Clean with whiting and sweet-oil, or prepared chalk and whiskey, rubbed on with flannel. Polish with a piece of soft buckskin, or a soft brush, made for that purpose.

METHOD FOR CLEANING FINE BLOCK TIN DISH COVERS, PATENT PEWTER, ETC.

Where the polish has gone off, let the articles be rubbed over the outside with a little sweet-oil on a piece of soft linen cloth; then clean it off with dry, pure whiting, quite free from sand, on linen cloths. The inside should be rubbed with rags moistened in wet whiting, but without a drop of oil. Always wiping these articles dry when brought from the table; and keeping them free from steam, or other dampness, greatly diminishes the trouble of cleaning them.

TO CLEAN BRITANNIA WARE.

Mix together some yellow soap, sweet-oil, and enough rum or whiskey to make the preparation the consistency of thick cream. Dip into it a soft sponge, and rub it evenly and quickly on the article; then wipe it off, and polish with a piece of silk or buckskin.

ANOTHER METHOD.

Britannia ware should be first rubbed gently with a woollen cloth and sweet-oil; then washed in warm suds, and rubbed with soft leather and whiting. Thus treated, it will retain its beauty to the last.

TO REMOVE MEDICINE STAINS FROM SILVER.

Silver spoons frequently become discolored by using them in taking medicine. These stains, even that of muriate of iron, may be removed by rubbing the spoon with sulphuric acid, and afterwards washing it off in soap-suds; then cleaning the spoon in the usual manner.

A FINE PLATE MIXTURE.

Take one pound of the best whiting, rub it to a fine powder, and sift it. Mix together four ounces of spirits of turpentine; two ounces of spirits of wine; one ounce of spirits of camphor; and half an ounce of hartshorn. Then add the whiting gradually to the liquid, stirring in a little at a time, and mixing the whole thoroughly till it is of the consistency of cream: put it into a very close vessel, and cork tightly, tying down a leather over the cork. To use the mixture, pour out a sufficient quantity, and with a soft, clean sponge cover the silver with it, so as to give it a coat like white-wash. Set it aside for ten minutes or more, till the paste has dried into a powder; then polish, first with a buckskin, and afterwards with a silk handkerchief. It will be found convenient to keep this mixture always ready for use, as it makes plate look beautifully new.

CEMENT FOR MENDING BROKEN CHINA OR GLASSWARE.

Mix half a pint of skimmed milk with an equal quantity of vinegar, so as to coagulate the milk. Separate the curd from the whey, and mix the former with the whites of four or five eggs, after beating them up well. The mixture of these two substances being complete, add sifted quicklime, and make the whole into a thick paste of the consistence of putty. If this be carefully applied to broken bodies, or to fissures of any kind, and dried properly, it resists fire and water.

ANOTHER REMEDY.

Pound burned oyster-shells, sift the powder through a very fine sieve, and grind it on a painter's stone till it becomes very fine; then take the whites of several eggs, according to the quantity of powder, beat them well, and having mixed them with it, form the whole into a kind of paste; join the pieces of china or glass, press them together for seven or eight minutes, and the united parts will stand heat and water, and will not come apart if they should fall to the ground.

CHINESE METHOD OF MENDING CHINA.

Take a piece of flint glass, beat it to a fine powder, and grind it with the white of an egg; this mixture joins china without riveting, so that no art can break it in the same place. The composition is to be ground extremely fine on a painter's stone.

HOW TO GET A TIGHT RING OFF A FINGER.

Thread a needle, flat in the eye, with a strong thread, pass the head of the needle, with care, under the ring, and pull the thread through a few inches towards the hand; wrap the long end of the thread tightly round the finger, regularly all down to the nail, to reduce its size. Then lay hold of the short end and unwind it. The thread passing against the ring, will gradually remove it from the finger. This never-failing method will remove the tightest ring without difficulty, however much swollen the finger may be.

TO EXTRACT A GLASS STOPPER.

Take a large strip of wool; pass it once around the neck of the bottle; attach one end of this to a board, or some fixed object; hold the other, and then seesaw the bottle along it. The friction will soon heat the neck of the bottle, and by the heat the neck will expand sufficiently to allow of the stopper being extracted.

TO REMOVE PANES OF GLASS.

Put soft soap on the putty for a few hours, and it becomes as soft as if just put on, though the putty had become as hard as a stone.

TO MAKE PASTE.

Putting acetate or sugar of lead into it, instead of the old way of mixing it with alum, keeps it free from mold, clear, and quite moist for months together.

TO CLEAN PAINT THAT IS NOT VARNISHED.

Put upon a plate some of the best whiting; have ready some clear, warm water, and a piece of flannel, which dip into the water, and squeeze nearly dry; then take as much whiting as will adhere to it; apply it to the paint, when a little rubbing will instantly remove any dirt or grease. Wash well off with water, and rub it dry with a soft cloth. Paint thus cleansed looks equal to new, and without doing the least injury to the most delicate color. It will preserve the paint much longer than if cleaned with soap, and it does not require more than half the time usually occupied in cleaning.

A WASH TO CLEAN PICTURES.

Make a ley with clear water and wood-ashes; in this dip a sponge, and rub the picture over, and it cleanses it perfectly. The same may be done with chamber-ley alone, or with white wine.

TO REVIVE OLD WRITINGS, WHICH ARE ALMOST DEFACED.

Boil gall-nuts into wine; steep a sponge into that liquor; then pass it on the lines of the old writing, and all the letters which were almost undecipherable will appear as fresh as when newly done.

TO PREVENT MOLDING IN BOOKS, INK, PASTE, AND LEATHER.

Collectors of books will not be sorry to learn that a few drops of oil of lavender will insure their libraries from this pest. A single drop of the same oil will prevent a pint of ink from molding any length of time. Paste may be kept from mold entirely by its addition; and leather is also effectually secured from injury by the same agency.

TO CLEAN KNIVES AND FORKS.

Procure a smooth board, cover it with leather; melt a sufficient quantity of mutton suet, and put it hot upon the leather with a piece of flannel. Then take two pieces of soft Bath brick, and rub them one against the other over the leather till it is covered with the powder, which rub in until no grease comes through when a knife is passed over the leather, which may be easily known by the knife's keeping its polish.

TO KEEP UP SASH WINDOWS.

This is performed by means of cork, in the simplest manner, and with scarcely any expense. Bore three or four holes in the sides of the sash, into which insert common bottle-corks, projecting about the sixteenth part of an inch. These will press against the frames, along the usual grooves, and by their elasticity support the sash at any height which may be required.

COMPOSITION FOR RAZORS.

Common candle-snuff, clear of grit, spread on a razor-strop, produces the best edge, in the shortest time, of anything ever tried. The coat should be spread with a knife, not too thick, and will last several months; first rub the strap with a little clean tallow.

WOOD POLISHING.

The Persians have introduced an entirely new mode of polishing, which is to wood precisely what plating is to metal. Water may be spilled on it without staining, and it resists scratching the same as marble. The receipt is as follows: —

To one pint of spirits of wine, add half an ounce of gum shellac, and half an ounce of gum sandrick, placing it over a gentle heat, and frequently agitating it until the gums are dissolved, when it is fit for use.

Make a roller of list, put a little of the polish upon it, and cover that with a soft linen rag, which must be slightly touched with cold-drawn linseed-oil. Rub them in the wood, in a circular direction, not covering too large a space at a time, till the pores are sufficiently filled up. After this, rub in the same manner spirits of wine with a small portion of the polish added to it, and a most brilliant polish will be produced. If the outside has been previously polished with wax, it will be necessary to clean it off with glass paper.

POLISH FOR DINING TABLES.

Rub them with cold-drawn linseed-oil, thus:—Put a little in the middle of a table, and then with a piece of linen (never use woollen) cloth, rub it well all over the table; then take another piece of linen, and rub it for ten minutes; then rub it quite dry with another cloth. This must be done every day for several months, when you will find your mahogany acquire a permanent and beautiful lustre, unattainable by any other means, and equal to the finest French polish; and if the table is covered with the table-cloth only, the hottest dishes will make no impression upon it. When once this polish is produced, it will only require dry rubbing, with a linen cloth, for about ten minutes, twice in a week, to preserve it in the highest perfection.

COMPOSITION FOR MAKING COMMON WOOD RESEMBLE MAHOGANY.

This will make any species of wood, of a close grain, so nearly to resemble mahogany in the nature, density, and polish, that the most accurate judges are incapable of distinguishing between this happy imitation and the native produce. The first operation, as now practised in France, is to plane the surface, so as to render it perfectly smooth; the wood is then to be rubbed with diluted nitrous acid, which prepares it for the materials subsequently to be applied. Afterward one ounce and a half of dragon's blood, dissolved in a pint of spirits of wine, and one-third of that quantity of carbonate of soda, are to be mixed together and filtered, and the liquid in this state is to be rubbed, or rather laid upon the wood with a soft brush. This process is repeated, with very little alteration; and in a short interval afterward the wood possesses the external appearance of mahogany; when this application has been properly made, the surface will resemble an artificial mirror: but if the polish become less brilliant, by rubbing it with a little cold-drawn linseed-oil, the wood will be restored to its former brilliancy.

USEFUL COMPOSITION.

To prevent friction, and facilitate the running of machinery, the best thing in use is said to be grease, eight parts, to two parts of black-lead, intimately mixed.

TO PREVENT THE SMOKING OF A LAMP.

Soak the wick in strong vinegar, and dry it well before you use it; it will then burn well, and give much satisfaction for the trifling trouble in preparing it.

SMOKY CHIMNEYS.

It has been clearly demonstrated by science and practical experiments that this great drawback upon domestic comfort is remedied by a simple process, viz., a slight, but continued enlargement, commencing at the bottom of the flue, and extending to the top. This is sure to produce a draught, and it is presumed that in most instances of defective chimneys, inattention to this simple rule, in the original construction would be found to be the cause of the evil.

TO PREVENT SOOT FROM ACCUMULATING IN CHIMNEYS.

Instead of plastering the inside of chimneys in the usual way, take mortar made with one peck of salt to each bushel of lime, adding as much sand and lime as will render it fit to work, and then lay on a thick coat. If the chimney has no offsets for the soot to lodge on, it will continue perfectly clear and free from all danger of taking fire.

COMPOSITION TO DEFEND THE ROOF OF A HOUSE FROM THE WEATHER AND FIRE.

Take one measure of fine sand, two measures of wood-ashes well sifted, three of slackened lime ground up with oil; lay this on with a painter's brush — first coat thin, and second thick. This mixture adheres so strongly to a board that it resists an iron tool, and the operation of fire.

COMPOSITION FOR PRESERVING FARMERS' UTENSILS.

Put three-fourths of a pound of resin into an iron kettle, with three gallons of train-oil, and three or four rolls of brimstone; when they are melted and become thin, add as much Spanish brown, or any other color you choose, ground up in oil in the usual way, as will give the color you desire; then lay on a thin coat with a brush, and when dry lay on another. This will preserve barrows, plows, carts, wagons, yokes, gate-posts, weather-boards, shingles, &c., many years from the effects of the weather.

COMPOSITION FOR PRESERVING HARNESS.

The following is a method of preserving leather, harness, and traces, engine hose, boots, and shoes, cording, cart and wagon covers, stack cloths, &c., in the most effectual manner: — Take of neatsfoot-oil one quart; beeswax, cut small, one ounce; oil of tar half a pound; and after simmering the neatsfoot-oil and wax a little in a pipkin, the oil of tar must be added; when, after a gentle simmering again for a few minutes, stirring it the whole time with a stick, the mixture will be finished, though an ounce of naphtha added would be a considerable improvement. It is used precisely as oil would be applied, and where it may be required to soften old and hardened leather, a sponging with hot water first, is advisable, and the liquid should be driven in before the fire. Leather, or cordage, dressed with this liquid, never rots, hardens, nor grows moldy.

When it is desirable to render leather water-proof, the ounce of naphtha proposed to be added should have a drachm of India-rubber dissolved in it. Naphtha is highly inflammable, and therefore should be kept from the fire and candle, and added after the mixture is taken from the fire.

COMPOSITION FOR PRESERVING BOOTS AND SHOES.

The receipt is as follows, and is to be used for the "uppers" only: — One half-pint neat's-foot oil, one ounce beeswax, one ounce spirits turpentine, one ounce tar, one half-ounce Burgundy pitch, to be slowly melted together, and well incorporated by stirring, taking care not to set the mass on fire, as the articles are all highly inflammable. The boots being damp, the composition is to be spread on with a small brush, taking care to cover the seams well, and then be allowed to dry; the application to be renewed until the leather is saturated.

For the soles, tar alone is the best application, to be put on while hot, the boots also having been by the fire, so that the soles are quite warm; if there is no grease, or other foreign matter, on the soles, three or four, or sometimes more, coats will sink into the leather; it must also be used until the soles are completely saturated. The trouble of preparing boots after the above directions is very trifling; and any one once having tried it, and experienced the comfort of being all day in the snow and slush, without having wet feet, will never fail to continue the use of it.

COMPOSITION TO RENDER SHOES WATER-TIGHT

One pint of drying oil, two ounces of yellow wax, two ounces of turpentine, half an ounce Burgundy pitch, melted carefully over a slow fire. If new shoes are rubbed carefully with this mixture, either in the sunshine or at some distance from the fire, with a sponge or soft brush, and the operation is repeated as often as they become dry, till the leather is fully saturated, they will be impervious to the wet, and will wear much longer, as well as acquire a softness and pliability that will prevent the leather from shrivelling.

Shoes or boots prepared as above ought not to be worn until perfectly dry and elastic, otherwise their durability would rather be prevented than increased.

BLACKING,

Which, when on the boots or shoes, can be rubbed with a cambric handkerchief, without soiling it in the least, and will assume the same lustre, after being plunged in water, as before: —

Quarter of a pound of ivory-black, one ounce of sweet-oil, one ounce spirits of lavender, one ounce oil of vitriol, two ounces sugar-candy, three pints best vinegar, or stale beer, and juice of two lemons.

The ivory-black and sweet-oil are to be well mixed in a mortar, the sugar-candy to be pounded, the vitriol to be put in a glass of water, and allowed to stand till cold. The spirits of lavender and oil of vitriol are not to be put in until all the other ingredients have been well mixed.

ANOTHER.

The following are said to be the materials of which Day & Martin's blacking is made: —

To one pound of ivory-black, in which has been mixed half an ounce of oil of vitriol and one ounce of sweet-oil, add one pound of pulverized loaf-sugar. Mix the whole with a gallon of vinegar, and let it stand three days, when it is fit for use.

It should be stirred often, and kept from the air to prevent evaporation. The cost of a gallon of this blacking is seventy-five cents, and is retailed at the stores at the rate of four dollars.

JAPAN COPAL VARNISH.

One ounce gum-copal, one ounce gum Arabic, one ounce gum tragacanth, four ounces gum shellac, and one-quarter of an ounce of gum myrrh; pound it fine, and put it in a quart of alcohol. Let it stand for half an hour; after that, the composition is fit for use.

For coloring red, one-quarter of an ounce of Sanders yellow, one-quarter of a pound of turmeric. To color black, one-quarter of an ounce of lamp-black.

Wood may be made any color, and when dry, this varnish will give it the gloss.

The best material for black color is the oil varnish, which may be obtained at any drug-store. To prepare the work for varnishing, oil it completely with linseed-oil, put on with a sponge.

How to apply the Varnish.—Absorb with a sponge a sufficient quantity to varnish the piece of work which is to be finished (three or four tablespoonsful is sufficient for a sideboard); over the sponge you must put a cotton or linen cloth; then apply to the cloth a little linseed-oil, which may be frequently repeated while varnishing. The varnish dries as it is applied to the wood, and at the same time gives the tint or shade required, if the coloring material is mixed with it.

The varnish may be mixed with the coloring material, and the varnish and coloring all done at the same time, or the coloring may be given first; after which the varnish may be applied. If the varnishing and coloring are to be performed at the same time, a sufficient quantity of varnish and coloring matter must be mixed together to varnish the work to be finished. If, however, it is desirable to varnish and color separately, the color should be laid on first, and when dry the varnish may be laid on as above directed.

TO MAKE JAPANESE CEMENT, OR RICE GLUE.

This cement is made by mixing rice-flour intimately with cold water, and then gently boiling it. It is beautifully white, and dries almost transparent. Papers pasted together by means of this cement will sooner separate in their own substance than at the joining, which makes it extremely useful in the preparation of curious paper articles, as tea-trays, ladies' dressing-boxes, and other articles which require layers of paper to be cemented together. It is, in every respect, preferable to common paste made with wheat flour, for almost every purpose to which that article is usually applied. It answers, in particular, for pasting into books the copies of writings taken off by copying-machines, or insized silver paper. With this composition, made with a comparatively small quantity of water, that it may have a consistence similar to that of plastic clay, models, busts, stays, and the like, may be formed when dry. The articles made of it are susceptible of a very high polish. They are also very durable.

TO MAKE A BEAUTIFUL AND LASTING WHITEWASH.

Take a quarter of a peck of unslacked lime, and pour on it a kettle of boiling water; while the lime is slacking, add half a gallon of stale chamber-ley; when the lime is perfectly slacked, dilute it with water to the proper consistence, and add to this mixture one-quarter of an ounce of Prussian blue. This will give you a beautiful and lasting wash, that will neither peel off nor turn yellow, and will look nearly as well as white paint. By increasing the quantity of blue, you may make either a pale or a dark blue, as best suits your taste: or, if you prefer it, by adding yellow or red ochre, you may impart either of these tints to your wash.

TO MAKE A BRILLIANT STUCCO WHITEWASH FOR BUILDINGS, INSIDE OR OUT.

Add one-quarter of a pound of whiting, or burned alum pulverized; one pound of loaf-sugar; three quarts of rice-flour, made into a thin and well-boiled paste; one pound of the cleanest glue, dissolved in the same way as by cabinet-makers. This mixture may be put on cold within doors, but hot outside. This preparation will be as brilliant as plaster of Paris, and retain its brilliancy for many years.

TO MAKE A CHEAP PAINT, OR WHITEWASH.

Take two quarts of skimmed-milk, two ounces of fresh slacked lime, and five pounds of whiting. Put the lime into a stone vessel, pour upon it a sufficient quantity of milk to make a mixture resembling cream; then add the remainder of the milk. When this is done, crumble and spread the whiting on the surface of the fluid, in which it will gradually sink. It must, after all the whiting has been precipitated, be well stirred, or ground as you would other paint, when it will be fit for use. By the addition of any coloring matter, you may make it to suit your fancy. It should be put on with a paint-brush, and when dry a second coat should be given. The quantity above mentioned is sufficient for twenty-seven yards.

ANOTHER.

Take one bushel of lime, and slack it with cold water; when well slacked, add to it twenty pounds of Spanish whiting, seventeen pounds of salt, and twelve pounds of sugar. Strain this mixture through a wire sieve, and it will be fit for use after reducing it with cold water. This is intended for the outside of a building, where it is exposed to all weather. In order to give a good color, three coats are necessary on brick, and two on wood. It may be laid on with a whitewash brush. Each coat must have a sufficient time to dry before the next is applied.

For painting inside walls, take one bushel of unslacked lime, three pounds of sugar, five pounds of salt; prepare as above, and apply with a brush. It is well calculated to preserve brick walls; and is far preferable to oil paint. This paint will preserve rough boards longer than dressing them, and covering them with oil paint. You can make any color you please. For straw color, use yellow ochre instead of whiting; for lemon color, ochre and chrome yellow; for lead and slate color, lampblack; for blue, indigo; for green, chrome green. These different kinds of paints will not cost one-fourth as much as oil paints, including the putting on.

A CHEAP WHITE PAINT.

One pound of unslacked lime, one pound of Spanish whiting, one gallon of sweet milk, one gallon of flaxseed oil, one tablespoonful of lime; pour on the lime sufficient water to slack it, and while the lime is slacking, pour in the oil; add the whiting and salt, and then pour on the milk, and stir it well.

A CHEAP GREEN PAINT.

Take four pounds of Roman vitriol, and pour upon it a tea-kettleful of boiling water. When the vitriol is dissolved, add two pounds of pearlash, and stir the mixture well with a stick until the effervescence ceases; then add a quarter of a pound of pulverized yellow arsenic, and stir the whole together. Lay it on with a paint-brush, and if the wall has not been painted, two or three coats will be necessary. If a pea-green be required, put on less; and if an apple-green, more of the yellow arsenic.

The cost of this paint is less than one-fourth of oil color, and the beauty far superior.

PERMANENT INK FOR MARKING LINEN.

This useful ink is composed of nitrate of silver (lunar caustic), and tincture or infusion of galls, in the proportions of one drachm of the former, in a dry state, to two drachms of the latter. The linen or cotton must be first soaked in the following liquid, viz: salt of tartar, one ounce, dissolved in one ounce and a half of water; and must be perfectly dry before any attempt is made to write upon it.

MARKING OR DURABLE INK.

Take six cents' worth of lunar caustic, and having put it into an ounce vial full of vinegar, cork it tight and hang it in the sun. In a couple of days it will be fit for use. To make the preparation for the above, take a lump of pearlash of the size of a chestnut, and dissolve it in a gill of rain-water. The part of the muslin or linen to be written upon, is to be wet with the preparation, and dried and glazed with a warm flat-iron: immediately after which, it is ready for marking.

TO MAKE BLACK INK.

In three pints of vinegar, let three ounces of gall-nuts, one ounce powdered logwood, and one ounce green vitriol, be steeped half an hour; then add one half-ounce gum Arabic, and when the gum is dissolved, pass the whole mixture through a hair sieve.

IMPROVED COMPOSITION OF BLACK WRITING INK.

Take a gallon of soft water, and boil in it one pound of chips of logwood for about half an hour; then take the decoction from the fire, and pour it from off the chips, while boiling hot, on a pound of the best Aleppo galls, reduced to a fine powder, and two ounces of pomegranate peels. After having stirred them well together with a wooden spoon, or ladle, for some time, place them in the sunshine in summer, or within the warmth of the fire, if in winter, for three or four days, stirring the mixture as often as may be convenient; at the end of that time, add half a pound of green vitriol, powdered, and let the mixture remain four or five days more, stirring it frequently, and then add further four ounces gum Arabic, dissolved in a quart of boiling water; and after giving the ink some time to settle, strain it off from the dregs, and keep it well stopped for use.

If the ink be desired to shine more, the proportion of the pomegranate peel must be increased.

In order to secure this ink from growing moldy, a quarter of a pint of spirits of wine may be added;

but to prevent its containing any acid which may injure the ink, a little salt of tartar, or pearlash, should be added previously, and the spirits poured off from it.

FOR MAKING RED INK.

Infuse four ounces of ground Brazil-wood in one quart of vinegar for three days, then heat it to the boiling point, and keep it for an hour at that temperature; after which, it must be filtrated. While hot, dissolve in it one-third of an ounce of gum Arabic, and the same quantity of sugar, and of alum; allow it to cool, and put it into bottles well stopped. An ink of a still more beautiful shade may be made with a decoction of cochineal, to which ammonia is to be added.

HOW TO PREPARE PRINTER'S INK.

Take one pound of common turpentine, made with juniper and linseed-oil. Add to it one ounce of resin black, which is the smoke of it, and a sufficient quantity of oil of nuts.

Set this composition on the fire, and boil it to a good consistence. In the summer it must boil a little more than in winter, for in the summer the ink must be thicker, because the heat makes it more fluid.

FOR STOPPING A LEAK IN A CASK.

The best thing for stopping a leak in a cask is whiting beaten up with common yellow soap. If this mixture be well rubbed into the leak, it will be found to stop it after everything else has failed.

TO PRESERVE NAILS FROM RUSTING.

Take cut nails, and heat them pretty hot, but not red hot, in a fire-shovel over the fire, and then drop them into a glazed vessel containing train oil. They absorb a good deal of oil, and when thus prepared, never become rusty, and will last many years. Hinges and screws that are exposed to the weather would be equally benefited by such a treatment. The preparaiton of cut or wrought nails used in making board fences, or in any place where there is considerable exposure to the weather, in the manner recommended above, would be a decided improvement.

GREASE FOR WHEEL AXLES.

Thicken half a pint of melted grease with black-lead in powder, having previously thrown in and melted a lump of beeswax of the size of a small hickory-nut. Apply it to the hubs and axles before it hardens. In warm weather, use tallow instead of soft grease. Black-lead is sometimes gritty, that is, it contains sand, and such should be rejected. If tar has been previously applied to the hubs and axles, it ought to be carefully removed before the composition is applied; and until the pores of the wood become filled with the composition, it may escape from the boxes in that way, and render frequent examinations for the first few weeks necessary.

BROWNING STEEL OR IRON.

After a long series of experiments, Mr. Ettrich has discovered, and made known in a foreign journal, a process of procuring a permanent oxide, and then giving it a dark-brown or black color. The iron or steel of a rifle-barrel, for instance, must be well smoothed and polished, and all greasiness removed by chalk before browning commences. Then mix one part of nitric acid with one hundred parts of water, and, moistening a rag in this, apply it to the barrel. It is material that the rag should only be moistened, for if instead of damping the iron, the fluid streams over it, the browning will be imperfect and irregular. The barrel, after being wet, should be placed in a window on which the sun shines, for an hour or more; and when this process has been twice or thrice repeated, the superfluous rust must be removed by a scratch-brush, consisting of a quantity of fine wire tied up into a bundle. This process being repeated eight or ten times, the barrel will have acquired as perfect a brown as is usually given by gunsmiths; but to take away the rusty appearance that remains on the iron, it is browned or blacked, by dissolving one grain of nitrate of silver in five hundred of water, and applying this solution in the same way as the acid. The number of repetitions of nitrate of silver water will depend on the shade of blackness required, but from one to five will be sufficient: at each wetting with the nitrate, the barrel should be placed in the sunshine, to insure a dark color. The last process is to apply the scratch freely, though lightly, and then polish the whole down by beeswax. Mr. Ettrich found by experiment, after becoming acquainted with the process used by the trade, that his system of operation produced a much finer and darker brown than could be given by theirs, and is decidedly more simple and easy in being carried into effect.

PIG TROUGHS.

Take two pieces of board or plank, of the length that you wish your trough; put two of their edges together at right angles, and nail them strong; then take two pieces, something longer than the trough is wide, and nail upon the ends; then take some clay mortar and fill up the chinks to prevent its leaking, and it is done. The food settles down in the bottom of the trough, and the pig will lay his sharp under jaw into it completely, while the long ends prevent its being upset so easily as the old kind. Anybody who can saw a board off, or drive a nail, can make one. If you have no trough for your pig, just try your hand at making one on this plan.

FENCE POSTS.

An excellent method of rendering fence posts durable in the ground, consists, 1st. In peeling the posts, and in sawing and splitting them, if too large. 2d. In sticking them up under cover, at least one entire summer; and, 3d. In coating with hot tar about three feet of the but-ends, which are to be inserted in the ground; after which they are ready for use. We have no doubt that the advantages of this mode of preparation will more than remunerate for labor and expense. The best timber is obtained from trees which have stood a year, after they have been girdled and peeled.

FENCE POSTS—ANOTHER.

The durability of posts, used in making fences, is a matter of great importance to farmers, and will continue so as long as the present system of fencing is continued. We are informed that the Shakers of

Union Village have been in the habit of making oak posts as durable as locust, by a very simple and easy process. This is merely to bore a hole in that part of the post which will be just at the surface of the earth, with such a slope as will carry it just below the surface, and fill it with salt. This, it is said, will preserve the timber from decaying for a long time; and, from the knowledge we have of the influence of salt in preserving ship-timber, when treated in a similar manner, we have no doubt of its being an excellent method.

MEASURING CORN.

Having previously levelled the corn in the house, so that it will be of equal depth throughout, ascertain the length, depth, and breadth of the bulk; multiply these dimensions together, and their products by four; then cut off one figure from the right of the last product: this will give so many bushels, and decimal bushels of shelled corn. If it be required to find the quantity of corn in the ears, substitute 8 for 4, and cut off one figure as before.

Example. — In a bulk of corn in the ears, measuring twelve feet long, eleven feet broad, and six feet deep, there will be 316 bushels, and eight-tenths of a bushel of shelled corn; or 633 bushels of ears, as follows:—

	12	12
	11	11
	132	132
	6	6
	792	792
	4	8
Shell corn,	316.8	633.6 ears.

The decimal 4 is used when the object is to find the quantity in shelled corn, because that decimal is half of the decimal, and it requires two bushels of ears to make one of shelled corn. In using these rules, a half-bushel should be added for every hundred, that amount of error resulting from the substitution of the decimals.

TO CALCULATE INTEREST.

A short and simple method of calculating interest at six per cent. per annum.

Rule.—Multiply the principal by half the number of months.

Example.—What is the interest of forty dollars for twelve months?

$40 the principal.
6 half the number of months.

$2.40 answer.

Example.—What is the interest of forty dollars for seven months?

$40
$3\frac{1}{2}$

1.20
20

$1.40 *answer.*

ANOTHER METHOD OF COMPUTING INTEREST.

An accurate and easy way to calculate interest is to multiply the sum by the number of days; that product being divided by 6 will give the interest in mills;

then strike off the right-hand figure, and the remainder will be in cents.

Example. 1250 dollars.
80 days.

Divide by 6)100000

Interest at 6 per cent. for 80 days, $16.66,7

If 7 per cent. is required, add one-sixth more to the interest.

When the amount to be multiplied has a fraction, it is usual to drop it if under 50 cents, or count it another dollar if over.

Each whole month should be reckoned as 30 days.

TO KILL WASPS OR YELLOW JACKETS.

When a wasp's nest is found, take about half a pint of tar in a pitch ladle, and run part of it into a hole where the nest is; put the remainder of the tar round about the mouth of the hole, and the job is done. All the wasps that are in the nest are caught in their attempt to come out, and those that are out are caught in their attempt to go in, so that none escape. If the nest should be in a place where the tar will soon get dry, it may perhaps be better to put a little more tar round the hole the following day, as in general there are a great many of them which are out all night, and when the tar is dry it will not catch them. It is not necessary to dig out the nest, and the tar may be applied at any time of the day, even when the wasps are most busy.

Should the wasps build their nests any place out of the ground, they might easily be destroyed by smoking them well with brimstone after night.

IMPORTANT DISCOVERY; OR, HOW TO KILL CROWS WITH NEW ENGLAND RUM.

Soak some corn in a quantity of rum, until it is saturated therewith, and then spread it in a corn-field infested with crows. The crows will eat, become stupefied, and then may be easily killed.

TO PREVENT CROWS FROM PULLING UP CORN.

Soak seed-corn in a solution of Glauber salts, from twenty-four to forty-eight hours before planting, and no living animal, with the sense of taste, will eat it.

SCARE-CROWS.

The best scare-crows we have ever used, were bright sheets of tin suspended from poles, by wires; the poles of sufficient height, and in sufficient numbers, to be seen all over the field. Four or six, if judiciously placed, will effectually answer for a field of fifty acres. The mode of fixing them is this: cut a pole of sufficient height, trim off all the limbs but the upper ones; to the end of this limb attach, by a strong flexible wire, a sheet of tin, and plant the pole, thus provided, firmly in the ground, on the destined spot. The limb left at the top, should project horizontally far enough to allow full play to the tin. Thus attached, the slightest breeze gives motion to the tin, and consequently causes a reflection so sudden as to effectually frighten off the crows, or other birds addicted to picking up the corn.

ESTIMATING THE WEIGHT OF CATTLE.

In a country like ours, where great numbers of cattle are annually bought and sold, under circumstances which preclude the possibility of ascertaining their weight with positive accuracy, it must be desirable that some general rules, approximating to exactness, should be known, in order to prevent mistake on the part of the interested individuals. In England, two or three tables have been constructed by different individuals, founded on the length and girth of the animal, at certain points, and based on a vast number of experiments, most carefully made. To illustrate this matter, we have copied from an English work the figure and tables, as follows: —

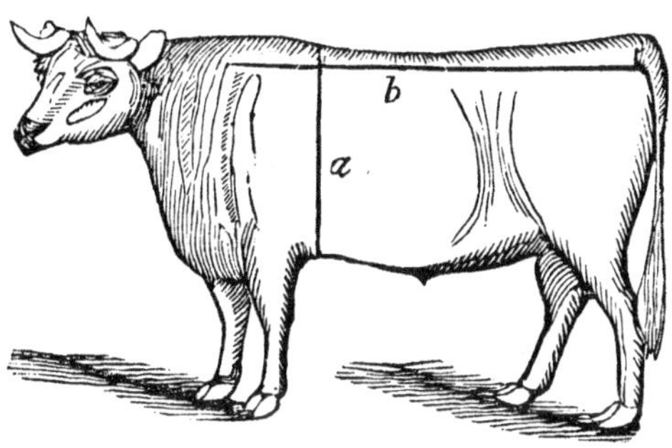

Girth.		*Length.*		*Renton's Table.*		*Cary's Table.*	
feet.	in.	feet.	in.	stone.	lb.	stone.	lb
5	0	3	6	21	0	21	0
		4	0	24	0	24	0
5	6	3	9	27	1	27	0
		4	0	34	4	34	7
6	0	4	6	38	8	38	11
		5	0	43	1	43	0
6	6	4	6	45	9	45	7
		4	9	48	0	48	0
7	0	5	6	64	6	64	7
		6	0	70	5	70	3
8	0	6	6	99	8	99	12
		7	0	107	5	107	6

The manner of taking the girth and length of an animal is as follows: — The girth is taken by passing a line just behind the shoulder-blade, and under the fore-legs (see line on the figure): this gives the circumference of the animal. The length is taken along the back, from the foremost corner of the blade-bone of the shoulder, in a straight line, to the hindmost point of the rump, or to that bone of the tail that plumbs the line with the hinder part of the buttock. These lines are then measured by the foot-rule, and the weight can readily be calculated from the tables. Some slight difference of weight may be traced in the tables, and also in another one, calculated by M. Derment: but the agreement is sufficiently close to show that no material error can exist. The tables, according to the English mode of reckoning, are calculated upon the stone of fourteen pounds, avoirdupois; thus, if the girth is six feet, and the length five feet, the weight will be forty-three stone, one pound, or six hundred and three pounds. Mr. Renton, in his "Grazier's Ready Reckoner," states that for a half-fattened ox, one stone in every twenty must be deducted; and when they are very fat, one-twentieth may be added. No tables can, however, be at all times implicitly relied upon, as there are many circumstances connected with the build of the animal, the mode of fattening, &c., that will influence the measurement, and consequently the weight. As a general guide, such tables must be useful to the farmer, or grazier, for whose use they are of course principally intended.

TO CURE SHEEP-SKINS WITH THE WOOL ON.

Take a spoonful of alum, and two of saltpeter; pulverize and mix well together, then sprinkle the powder on the inside of the skin, and lay the two insides together, leaving the wool outside. Then fold up the whole skin as tight as you can, and hang in a dry place. In two or three days, as soon as dry, take down, and scrape with a blunt knife till clean and supple; this completes the process, and makes a most excellent saddle-cover. If, when you kill the sheep, you treat the skins in this way, you can get more for them from the saddlers than you can for the wool and skin disposed of separately.

Other skins which you desire to cure with the fur or hair on, may be treated in the same way.

RECEIPTS FOR HOUSEKEEPERS.

New iron should be very gradually heated at first. After it has become inured to the heat, it is not as likely to crack.

It is a good plan to put new earthenware into cold water, and let it heat gradually until it boils, then cool again. Brown earthenware, in particular, may be toughened in this way. A handful of rye, or wheat bran, thrown in while it is boiling, will preserve the glazing, so that it will not be destroyed by acid or salt.

Clean a brass kettle, before using it for cooking, with salt and vinegar.

The oftener carpets are shaken, the longer they will wear. The dirt that collects under them grinds out the threads.

If you wish to preserve fine teeth, always clean them thoroughly after you have eaten your last meal at night.

Do not wrap knives and forks in woollens; wrap them in good strong paper. Steel is injured by lying in woollens.

Suet keeps good all the year round, if chopped and packed down in a stone jar, covered with molasses.

Barley-straw is the best kind for beds. Dry corn-husks, slit in shreds, are better than straw.

Brass and irons should be cleaned, done up in papers, and put in a dry place during the summer.

When molasses is used for cooking, it is a great improvement to boil and skim it before using. It takes out the unpleasant raw taste, and makes it almost as good as sugar. Where molasses is used much for cooking, it is well to prepare one or two gallons in this way at a time.

Never allow ashes to be taken up in wood, or put into wood. Always have your matches and lamp ready for use in case of sudden alarm. Have important papers together, where you can lay your hands on them at once in case of fire.

Use hard soap to wash your clothes, and soft to wash your floors. Soft soap is so slippery that it wastes a good deal in washing clothes.

It is easy to have a supply of horse-radish all winter. Have a quantity grated while the root is in perfection, put it in bottles, fill them with vinegar, and keep them corked tight.

Woolen goods should be washed in very hot water, and as soon as the article is cleansed, immerse it in cold water; let it be wrung, and hung up to dry.

IMPROVED METHOD OF ROASTING COFFEE.

Coffee should be roasted but a short time before it is required for use. Attend to it carefully while it is roasting, that not a single grain may be burned, as a little neglect in this respect will make the whole bitter. Turn it about frequently, and let it all be well browned, but not black.

TO MAKE GOOD COFFEE OUT OF RYE.

The rye is to be well cleaned, and then boiled till soft; but care is to be taken that it does not burst. It is afterward to be dried in the sun, or in an oven, and then burnt like coffee; and, when ground, it is fit for use.

THE END.

INDEX.

THE END.

RECOMMENDATIONS OF "THE SOUTHERN GARDENER."

This is the third edition of a very useful work, by Mrs. Mary L. Edgeworth, who dedicates the volume to Mrs. E. Thornton, of Camden, S. C. It is eminently calculated for general use in the Southern States, where it will no doubt be very extensively circulated, especially as several valuable additions are now made to the original compilation. The directions for gardening were written by Mr. P. Thornton, of Camden, S. C., and Mrs. Edgeworth resides at Fort Valley, in Georgia —both places being located in the midst of a fertile soil and salubrious climate. Not only in the cultivation of the earth are the pages before us a valuable guide, but there are also directions for the dairy, veterinary receipts, cookery, medical, and miscellaneous items of all kinds. —*Pennsylvania Inquirer.*

The author aims to give the purchaser the full worth of his money. The receipts seem to be well selected, and we presume have the advantage of having been experimentally tested Most of such hand-books have special reference to the wants of the Northern and Middle States, and hence have failed, to some extent, to meet the demands of the South. The author, who is a Georgian, being familiar with the Southern climate, products, and tastes, has endeavored to adapt her receipts to that region. We commend the volume to the attention of our Southern readers especially, and doubt not they will find it a useful help on the farm and in the family. —*Philada. Presbyterian.*

This work contains valuable information, original and otherwise, on all subjects connected with domestic and rural affairs, gardening, cookery, beverages, dairy, medical, veterinary, and miscellaneous. Third edition. Revised and corrected by Mrs. Mary L. Edgeworth. The fact that a third edition of this work has been called for, is a presumptive proof of its excellence. To the present edition many original and selected receipts have been added—all of which, we are informed, together with those in the former editions, have been thoroughly tested. — *Godey's Lady's Book.*

We do not know which to admire most, the easy style which the authoress adopts, or the excellent arrangement and usefulness of the work. There is a happy avoidance of technicalities truly refreshing. The reader will gather from its pages many useful, practical lessons in gardening, cookery, etc.; but not the least valuable feature of the work is its medical department. We cheerfully commend the work to the favorable consideration of our readers, and hope they will avail themselves of the opportunity of securing a copy. — *Cartersville (Ga.) Express.*

It is a very handsome book of 478 pages, by a Southern lady, who has bestowed great care on the present edition, which, although issued but six weeks since, is nearly sold out. The gardening part of it was written by Mr. Phineas Thornton, of Camden, S. C. — a most experienced and intelligent gardener. It was written expressly for this work. —*Salisbury (N. C.) Watchman.*

After examining a copy of the third edition of this work, we find it contains a vast fund of information for the gardener and housekeeper. The work is in every way worthy of patronage. — *Cassville Standard.*

www.ingramcontent.com/pod-product-compliance
Lightning Source LLC
LaVergne TN
LVHW052216200926
848481LV00001B/130
9781425550998